MW01075798

Spanish for Pediatric Medicine

A Practical Communication Guide

by
Edward Machtinger, MD
Peter Andrija Nigrović, MD

edited by
Janice A. Lowe, MD

American Academy
of Pediatrics

DEDICATED TO THE HEALTH OF ALL CHILDREN™

Final Editing of Spanish Translation
by
Eduardo Budge, MD, and María García de Budge

First Edition — 1997, revised 2003

Library of Congress Control Number: 2002107236

ISBN: 1-58110-091-4

MA0210

The recommendations in this publication do not indicate an exclusive course of treatment or serve as a standard of medical care. Variations, taking into account individual circumstances, may be appropriate.

Statements and opinions expressed are those of the authors and not necessarily those of the American Academy of Pediatrics.

9-75/0802

Introduction

This guide was designed to enhance communication between health care professionals and their Spanish-speaking patients. It is not comprehensive; the use of professional interpreters is always ideal. Rather, the guide is a quick reference to help identify and explore medical problems in the setting of well-child care, sick visits, and the emergency room until more formal interpretation services can be arranged. The result, we hope, will be a more satisfying clinical encounter for all involved.

The guide assumes some familiarity with Spanish. For practicality, most Spanish questions in this book are phrased using the verb form appropriate both to *él/ella* and the formal *usted*. For the English questions, we have written *he/she/you*. The questions as they are written can be posed equally to parents about their children and to the children themselves. Those with greater proficiency in Spanish may wish to change the verb to the informal *tú* form when addressing children. We recognize that in English, the verb forms for the second and third person are not the same; however, to simplify the use of the guide, we have not written out both forms.

Spoken Spanish varies considerably by region. We have tried to select vocabulary broadly recognized across the Americas, but a few blank looks will be unavoidable.

Request for Comments

A note to our readers:

The authors and the American Academy of Pediatrics are interested in your reactions to and use of this edition. Please send us your comments and suggestions for future editions of this work.

Comments may be addressed to:
Department of Marketing and Publications
American Academy of Pediatrics
141 Northwest Point Blvd
PO Box 927
Elk Grove Village, IL 60009-0927

Acknowledgment

We are deeply indebted to Eduardo Budge, MD, and María García de Budge for their careful review and expert advice in the final editing of the Spanish translations.

We wish to thank Marylena Estrada Leonardo, Gloria Ciccone, MD; Wanda Gonzalez, MD; and Victoria McEvoy, MD, for their editing and suggestions. We are grateful to Merylee Van Houten for administrative assistance and to Deb Cohan, MD; M. Sheila Desmond, MD; Patricia McArdle, EdD; Anne Sedlock, Service MGH; and the staff of the Chelsea Healthcare Center, Massachusetts General Hospital, for their support and generous assistance. We are also indebted to John Machtinger for his expert advice and generosity.

We wish to thank the staff of the AAP Department of Marketing and Publications for their work on this project. We are also grateful to Rosario Gonzalez-De Rivas, MD, for her review of the manual.

And, finally, we would like to thank our families and friends for their love and patience during our many hours of work on this project. Special thanks to Paul Wise, MD, MPH; Jeff Schulden; Robert Landaw, MD; Yorke Rhodes, MD; and Marylena Estrada Leonardo for their faith in our project and their unwavering support.

Table of Contents

Target Systems

Emergency Department Visit

Special Issues

Additional Words and Phrases

Appendix

Index

Common Expressions

Greetings	**Saludos**
Hello.	Hola.
Good morning, good afternoon, good evening.	Buenos días, buenas tardes, buenas noches.
Do you speak English?	¿Habla usted inglés?
How are you? Fine, thank you.	¿Cómo está usted? Bien, gracias.
I am a doctor, medical student, nurse.	Soy médico, estudiante de medicina, enfermero/a.
I work with_____.	Trabajo con_____.
Dr _____ is not here today.	El doctor/la doctora _____ no está hoy.
Please come with me.	Pase conmigo, por favor. (Pase adelante, por favor.)
Please have a seat.	Siéntese, por favor.
Please wait here for a moment.	Espere aquí un momento, por favor.
Excuse me.	Perdóneme.
I am pleased to meet you.	Mucho gusto en conocerlo/a.
The pleasure is mine.	El gusto es mío.
I will talk with you later.	Hablaré con usted(es) después.
Good-bye.	Adiós.

Helpful Phrases	**Frases Útiles**
Please.	Por favor.
Thank you.	Gracias.
You're welcome (my pleasure).	De nada (con mucho gusto).
I don't speak Spanish very well.	No hablo español muy bien.
I'm sorry, I don't understand.	Lo siento, no entiendo.
Hold on, wait. (to interrupt rapid speech)	Espéreme. (or: Un momento, por favor.)
More slowly, please.	Más despacio, por favor.
Please repeat that. (Again, please?)	Repítame eso, por favor. (¿Otra vez, por favor?)
Tell me more about that.	Dígame más sobre eso.
Please try to answer with "yes" or "no."	Por favor, trate de contestar solamente "sí" o "no."
Can you understand me?	¿Me entiende?
Please wait while I get a translator.	Por favor, espere mientras consigo un intérprete.
I'll be right back.	Ahora vuelvo.
Excuse me.	Perdóneme.
I am sorry.	Lo siento.
Please give this to the: secretary, nurse, lab.	Por favor, dele esto al/a la: secretario/a, enfermero/a, laboratorio.
This is common, normal.	Esto es común, normal.
Do not worry.	No se preocupe.

This is worrisome.	Esto es preocupante.
Do you understand?	¿Entiende?
Do you have any questions?	¿Tiene alguna pregunta?

Terms of Endearment for Children

Terminos Cariñosos Para Niños

boy/girl	chico/a, muchacho/a
boy/girl (diminutive and affectionate)	chiquito/a, muchachito/a
cute baby boy/girl	chulo/a, (or: mi bello/a) nene/nena
doll (girls only)	muñeca
How precious! (infants)	¡Qué precioso/a!
How handsome, pretty, beautiful!	¡Qué guapo/a, lindo/a!
How big!	¡Qué grande!
What a pretty dress/ handsome outfit!	¡Qué vestido/traje más precioso!
Your child is very beautiful/handsome.	Su niño/a es muy lindo/a/guapo.

General Visit

Initial History	Historia Inicial
Who is the patient?	¿Quién es el paciente?
What is his/her/your name?	¿Cómo se llama?
To child: What is your name?	¿Cómo te llamas?
How old is he/she/you?	¿Cuántos años tiene?
What is his/her/your birth date?	¿Cuál es su fecha de nacimiento?
Does he/she live with you?	¿Él/ella vive con usted?
What is your relationship to the patient?	¿Cuál es su relación con el paciente?
Who is his/her/your regular doctor?	¿Normalmente quién es su pediatra?
What brings you in today?	¿Qué les trae por acá? (¿Porque viene hoy?)
Is he/she/you here for a physical exam? Is it for school?	¿Está él/ella/usted aquí para un examen físico? ¿Es para la escuela?
Do you have any papers I need to fill out?	¿Trae algún papel que tengo que llenar?
Do you have a record of his/her immunizations?	¿Tiene algún registro de sus vacunas?

Past Medical History	Historia Médica Pasada

1. Medical History
2. Surgical History
3. Hospitalizations
4. Trauma
5. Medications
6. Allergies
7. Habits
8. Travel History
9. Immunizations
10. Birth History
11. Growth and Development
12. Nutrition

1. Medical History	1. Historia Médica
Does he/she/you have any (other) medical problems?	¿Tiene (otros) problemas médicos?
Has he/she/you ever had any serious illnesses? What? When?	¿Ha tenido alguna enfermedad seria? ¿Qué? ¿Cuándo?
Has he/she/you ever had:	¿Ha tenido alguna vez:
a heart murmur?	un soplo cardíaco?
tuberculosis?	tuberculosis?
exposure to anyone with TB?	contacto con alguien con TB?
a positive skin test for TB?	una prueba positiva de TB?
rheumatic fever?	fiebre reumática?

Have you ever been pregnant? How many times? When?	¿Has estado embarazada alguna vez? ¿Cuántas veces? ¿Cuándo?
Do you have any children? How many? How old?	¿Tienes hijos? ¿Cuántos? ¿De qué edades?
Have you ever had a miscarriage, abortion?	¿Has tenido alguna vez una pérdida, un aborto?

2. Surgical History

Has he/she/you ever had an operation? What for? When? Did he/she/you have any problems with the anesthesia?

2. Historia Quirúrgica

¿Ha tenido alguna vez una operación? ¿Para qué? ¿Cuándo? ¿Tuvo algún problema con la anestesia?

3. Hospitalizations

Has he/she/you ever been in the hospital? For what? When? For how long? Where?

3. Hospitalizaciones

¿Ha sido hospitalizado/a alguna vez? ¿Para qué? ¿Cuándo? ¿Por cuánto tiempo? ¿Dónde?

4. Trauma

Has he/she/you ever had any serious injuries?

Has he/she/you ever had any:

    stitches?
    broken bones?
    head injury?

    loss of consciousness?

4. Historia de Accidentes

¿Ha sufrido alguna herida seria?

¿Ha tenido alguna vez:

    puntos?
    huesos quebrados?
    herida/golpe en la cabeza?
    pérdida de consciencia?

5. Medications

Does he/she/you
take any medications?
Which ones?
What dose?
How many times
per day?

Are you taking the
birth control pill?

Does he/she/you use
any home remedy?
Other treatment
outside the medical
establishment?

6. Allergies

Is he/she/you allergic
to any medications?
Which ones?
What happened?
Rash, hives, difficulty
breathing?

Is he/she/you allergic
to any foods, animals,
pollens (hay fever)?

7. Habits

Do you smoke
cigarettes?
How many/day?
Since when?

Do you drink alcohol?
Beer, wine, liquor?
How much?

5. Medicaciones

¿Toma alguna
medicina?
¿Cuál?
¿En qué dosis?
¿Cuántas
veces al día?

¿Tomas la píldora
(anticonceptiva)?

¿Usa algún remedio
casero?
¿Otro tratamiento
fuera del sistema
médico?

6. Alergias

¿Tiene alergia a
alguna medicina?
¿Cuáles?
¿Qué le pasó?
¿Erupción, ronchas,
dificultad para respirar?

¿Tiene alergia a
alguna comida,
animal, polen (fiebre
del heno)?

7. Hábitos

¿Fumas
cigarrillos?
¿Cuántos al día?
¿Desde cuándo?

¿Tomas alcohol?
¿Cerveza, vino, licor?
¿Cuánto?

Do you use any drugs?	¿Usas alguna droga?
marijuana/grass	marihuana/hierba
cocaine	cocaína/coca
crack	crack
heroin	heroína
speed	anfetaminas/ estimulantes
LSD/acid	LSD/ácido
Have you ever used IV drugs?	¿Te has inyectado drogas alguna vez?
Ever shared needles (syringes)?	¿Has compartido agujas (jeringas) alguna vez?

8. Travel History / 8. Historia de Viajes

Where was he/she/you born?	¿Donde nació?
How long has he/she/you been in this country?	¿Por cuánto tiempo ha estado en los Estados Unidos?
Has he/she/you traveled outside the US recently? Where? When?	¿Viajó recientemente al extranjero? ¿Adónde? ¿Cuándo?
Have you had foreign visitors recently? From where?	¿Han recibido visitantes del extranjero recientemente? ¿De dónde?

9. Immunizations

Has he/she/you received all his/her/your immunizations? Do you have a record of them?

Has he/she/you ever had a reaction to a vaccine? Which vaccine? What happened?

10. Birth History

Were there any problems with the pregnancy?

Was your child born on time?

How many weeks early, late?

Did you deliver vaginally or by cesarean? Why? Were there any problems with the delivery?

Do you know the baby's Apgar scores?

How much did your baby weigh at birth?

9. Inmunizaciones

¿Ha recibido todas las vacunas que le tocan? ¿Tiene un registro de ellas?

¿Ha tenido alguna vez una reacción contra una vacuna? ¿Qué vacuna? ¿Qué le pasó?

10. Historia del Nacimiento

¿Hubo algún problema con el embarazo?

¿Nació su niño/a en el tiempo estipulado? ¿Cuántas semanas prematuro/a, tarde?

¿Fue un parto vaginal o por cesárea? ¿Por qué? ¿Hubo algún problema con el parto?

¿Sabe usted los números Apgar de su bebé?

¿Cuánto pesó al nacer?

How many days did your child spend in the hospital? Why?

¿Cuántos días pasó él/ella en el hospital? ¿Por qué?

Was the baby sick right after birth?

¿Estuvo enfermo/a su niño inmediatamente después de nacer?

11. Growth and Development

Has your child been growing normally?

What can your child do now?

Can your child do the same things as most children his/her age?

11. Crecimiento y Desarrollo

¿Crece normalmente su niño/a?

¿Qué puede hacer él/ella ahora?

¿Puede hacer lo mismo que la mayoría de niños de su edad?

12. Nutrition

Is your child eating well?
What is your child eating now?

Is he/she breast-feeding?
How often?

Is he/she drinking formula yet?
What type?
How many ounces per day?
Is he/she eating solid foods?
What kinds?
How much?

12. Nutrición

¿Come bien su niño/a?
¿Qué come su niño/a ahora?

¿Le da el pecho (todavía)?
¿Con qué frecuencia?

¿Toma fórmula (todavía)?
¿Qué tipo?
¿Cuántas onzas al día?
¿Come comida sólida?
¿De que tipo?
¿Cuánto?

Family History

Does he/she/you have
any brothers or sisters?
How many? How old are
they? Are they healthy?

Have any brothers or
sisters died?
Of what? At what age?

How old is his/her/your
father, mother, you?
Does he/she/you have
any medical problems?
Which?

To mother or father:
Do you have a doctor?
Do you need any help
finding a doctor?

Are his/her/your
grandparents alive?
What did he/she die of?
How old was he/she?
Do they have any
medical problems?

Do any other medical
problems run in the
family?
diabetes
heart disease
high blood pressure
cancer, of which type?
asthma
eczema
hay fever
alcoholism
drug addiction

Historia Familiar

¿Tiene hermanos o
hermanas?
¿Cuántos? ¿De qué
edades? ¿Están sanos?

¿Algún hermano o
hermana falleció?
¿De qué? ¿A qué edad?

¿Qué edad tiene el padre,
la madre, usted?
¿Tiene algún problema
médico?
¿Cuál?

¿Tiene usted un médico?
¿Necesita alguna ayuda
para obtener un médico?

¿Están vivos sus
abuelos?
¿De qué murió su abuelo/a?
¿Cuántos años tenía?
¿Tienen algún
problema médico?

¿Hay algún otro problema
médico que exista en la
familia?
diabetes
enfermedades cardíacas
presión alta
cáncer, de qué tipo?
asma
eczema
fiebre del heno
alcoholismo
drogadicción

obesity	obesidad
learning disability	problema de aprendizaje
slow development	retraso del desarrollo
problems with the	problemas con
skin	la piel
thyroid	la tiroides
heart	el corazón
lungs	los pulmones
stomach, intestines	el estómago, los intestinos
kidneys, urine	los riñones, la orina
blood	la sangre
nerves	los nervios
Family members	Miembros de la familia
parents	padres
mother	madre
father	padre
wife	esposa
husband	esposo
stepmother	madrastra
stepfather	padrastro
children	niños
daughter	hija
son	hijo
brother/sister	hermano/a
(older, younger)	(mayor, menor)
twin	gemelo/a
half brother/half sister	medio hermano/a
stepbrother/stepsister	hermanastro/a
grandfather/grandmother	abuelo/a
(father's/mother's side)	(paterno/a, materno/a)
uncle/aunt	tío/a
cousin	primo/a
nephew/niece	sobrino/a
mother-in-law	suegra
father-in-law	suegro
brother-in-law	cuñado
sister-in-law	cuñada

Social History (HEADSS)	Historia Social (HEADSS)
◆ **Home**	◆ **Hogar**
Where do you live?	¿Dónde viven?
Who lives at home with you?	¿Quién vive en casa con ustedes?
Does he/she/you have any problems at home?	¿Tiene problemas en casa?
Do you get along with your parents? Brothers? Sisters?	¿Te llevas bien con tus padres? ¿Hermanos? ¿Hermanas?
Does anyone at home drink alcohol? Too much?	¿Alguien en casa toma alcohol? ¿Demasiado?
Does anyone at home use drugs?	¿Alguien en casa usa drogas?
Do you always feel safe at home?	¿Siempre se siente seguro/a en casa?
Does anyone at home ever get violent?	¿Alguien en casa se ha puesto violento alguna vez?
How are things financially for the family?	¿Cómo están las finanzas en la casa?
Do you have enough food/formula?	¿Tienen ustedes suficiente comida/ fórmula?
Does anybody in the family work? What do they do?	¿Alguien en la familia trabaja? ¿Qué hacen?

Do you receive governmental assistance? WIC?	¿Reciben ayuda del gobierno? ¿WIC?
Do you have Medicaid? Health insurance?	¿Tienen Medicaid? ¿Seguro médico?

◆ **Education**

Are you in school? Where? In which grade?	¿Estás en la escuela? ¿Dónde? ¿En qué grado?
How do you like school?	¿Te gusta la escuela?
What is your favorite subject?	¿Cuál es tu materia favorita?
How are your grades?	¿Cómo son tus notas?
Do you receive any special help in school?	¿Recibes ayuda especial en la escuela?
Is there violence at school? Does it worry you?	¿Hay violencia en la escuela? ¿Te preocupa esto?

◆ **Activities**

◆ **Educación**

◆ **Actividades**

Do you have a best friend? Who? Other friends?	¿Tienes un/a mejor amigo/a? ¿Quién es? ¿Otros amigos?
What do you do for fun? After school?	¿Cómo te diviertes? ¿Después de la escuela?
Do you play sports? Which ones?	¿Haces deportes? ¿Cuáles?
How much television do you watch per day?	¿Cuánta televisión ves al día?
Do you work? Where? How often?	¿Trabajas? ¿Dónde? ¿Cuánto?

Do your friends carry weapons — knives, guns? How about you?	¿Cargan tus amigos armas — cuchillos, pistolas? ¿Y tú?

◆ Drugs

◆ Drogas

Do your friends drink alcohol?	¿Toman tus amigos alcohol?
Smoke cigarettes?	¿Fuman cigarrillos?
Use drugs?	¿Usan drogas?
How about you?	¿Y tú?
Have you ever injected drugs? What? How often?	¿Te has inyectado drogas alguna vez? ¿Cuál? ¿Con qué frecuencia?

◆ Sex

◆ Sexualidad

Is there anyone to whom you are sexually attracted?	¿Hay alguien a quien te sientas atraído/a sexualmente?
Are you attracted to men, women, or both?	¿Te gustan los hombres, las mujeres, o ambos?
Have you ever had questions about your sexual orientation?	¿Has tenido preguntas alguna vez sobre tu orientación sexual?
Do you have a boyfriend/girlfriend?	¿Tienes un/a novio/a?
Have you ever been sexually involved with anyone?	¿Has estado involucrado/a sexualmente con alguien alguna vez?
What type of sex do you have? Intercourse? Oral? Anal?	¿Qué tipo de sexo tienes? ¿Coito? ¿Oral? ¿Anal?

Do you want to become pregnant?	¿Quieres quedar embarazada?
Do you use any type of contraception? Which?	¿Usas algún tipo de anticonceptivo? ¿Cuál?
Condoms?	¿Preservativos (condones)?
Diaphragm?	¿Diafragma?
The pill?	¿La píldora?
Depo-Provera?	¿Depo-Provera?
Do you know how to use a condom?	¿Sabes cómo usar un condón?
Have you started menstruating yet? When?	¿Has empezado a menstruar ya? ¿Cuándo empezaste?
Are you regular? How long between periods?	¿Eres regular? ¿Cuánto tiempo entre períodos?
How many days are your periods?	¿Cuántos días duran los períodos?
Do you have painful cramps with your periods?	¿Tienes cólicos fuertes con los períodos?
Do the cramps keep you from doing regular activities? What do you do to relieve them?	¿Interfieren con tus actividades del día? ¿Qué haces para aliviarlos?
When did your last period start?	¿Cuándo empezó tu último período?
Do you have any children? How many?	¿Tienes hijos? ¿Cuántos?
Have you ever been pregnant? How many times? When?	¿Has estado embarazada alguna vez? ¿Cuántas veces? ¿Cuándo?

17

Have you ever had a miscarriage? An abortion?	¿Has tenido alguna vez una pérdida? ¿Un aborto?

◆ Suicide

How is your mood generally?

Does your mood go up and down often?

Do you ever feel very sad for a long time? About what?

Have you ever thought about killing yourself? Tell me about it.

How would you kill yourself?

Have you ever tried to kill yourself?

◆ Suicidio

¿Cómo está tu humor (estado de ánimo) generalmente?

¿Tienes cambios muy fuertes de humor?

¿Te sientes a veces muy triste por mucho tiempo? ¿Por qué?

¿Has pensado alguna vez en quitarte la vida? Cuéntame de esto.

¿Cómo te quitarías la vida?

¿Has tratado alguna vez de quitarte la vida?

Description of Pain

Has he/she/you been having pain?

Are you in pain now?

Where is the pain? Show me with one finger.

Does the pain go anywhere?

What is the pain like?

Descripción del Dolor

¿Ha estado teniendo dolor?

¿Tienes dolor ahora?

¿Dónde está el dolor? Muéstrame con el dedo.

¿Se va el dolor para algún lado?

¿Cómo es el dolor?

Is the pain:	¿Es el dolor:
mild, moderate, or severe?	leve, moderado, o severo?
constant, or does it come and go?	constante, o va y viene?
sharp, like a knife?	agudo, como de un cuchillo?
dull and aching?	sordo?
like pressure?	como presión?
burning?	ardiente?
gassy?	como gas?
crampy?	como calambre?
shooting/pricking?	punzante?
throbbing?	te pulsa?

When did the pain first start?	¿Cuándo empezó el dolor?
Did the pain start gradually or suddenly?	¿Empezó gradualmente o repentinamente?
Has the pain changed? Is the pain worse, better, or the same as before?	¿Ha cambiado el dolor? ¿Está el dolor peor, mejor, o igual que antes?
How often does he/she/you have the pain? All the time (without interruption)? How many times per day, per week, per month?	¿Con qué frecuencia tiene el dolor? ¿Todo el tiempo (sin interrupción)? ¿Cuántas veces al dia, a la semana, al mes?
How long does the pain last?	¿Cuánto dura el dolor?
Does anything make the pain better? Worse?	¿Hay algo que alivie el dolor? ¿Qué lo empeore?

Description of Pain (continued)

What brings on the pain?	¿Qué ocasiona el dolor?
food?	comida?
which ones?	cuáles?
how long afterwards?	cuánto tiempo después?
an empty stomach?	el estómago vacío?
bowel movements?	las evacuaciones?
urination?	el orinar?
a particular movement? Show me.	un movimiento en particular? Muéstrame.
exercise?	ejercicio?
(emotional) stress?	estrés (emocional)?
Do other symptoms come along with the pain?	¿Hay otros síntomas que acompañan el dolor?
Does the pain wake him/her/you up at night?	¿El dolor lo/la despierta en la noche?
Does he/she/you cry because of the pain?	¿Llora del dolor?
Has he/she/you taken anything for the pain? What? When? Did it help?	¿Ha tomado alguna medicina para el dolor? ¿Qué? ¿Cuándo? ¿Le ayudó?

Examination Instructions — Instrucciones Para el Exámen

Please take off all his/her/your clothes except for underwear/diaper.	Por favor, quítese toda la ropa excepto su ropa interior/pañal.
Here is an examination gown to wear.	Aquí hay una bata para que se ponga.

Please take off his/her/your	Por favor quítese
shirt	la camisa
pants	los pantalones
shoes and socks	zapatos y calcetines
underwear	la ropa interior
Please hold him/her in your arms for now.	Sosténgalo/la en sus brazos por ahora.
Hold (his/her arms, legs, head) like this.	Sostenga (sus brazos, sus piernas, su cabeza) así.
Put him/her on the examining table.	Póngalo/la sobre la camilla.
Please sit over here.	Siéntese aquí, por favor.

Note: the following instructions use the informal "tu" form.

Please	Por favor
lie down	acuéstate
sit up	siéntate
stand up	párate
turn over, around	voltéate
bend over and touch your toes	agáchate y toca la punta de tus pies
walk that way	camina hacia allá
now walk toward me	ahora camina hacia mí
stand on your (left, right) foot	párate en tu pie (izquierdo, derecho)
do this	haz esto
look at this	mirá esto

Examination Instructions (continued)

Watch my finger with your eyes.

Don't turn your head.

Open your mouth and say aah.

Stick out your tongue.

Breathe deeply (with your mouth open).

Hold your breath for a moment.

Relax your stomach.

How ticklish you are!

Does anything hurt?
Show me with your finger.
Does this hurt?
Tell me what hurts.

Instrucciones Para el Exámen (continuación)

Mira mi dedo con tus ojos.

No voltees la cabeza.

Abre la boca y dí aah.

Saca la lengua.

Respira profundo (con la boca abierta).

Contén tu respiración por un momento.

Relaja el estómago.

¡Qué cosquillas tienes!

¿Te duele algo?
Muéstrame con el dedo.
¿Te duele esto?
Dime lo que te duele.

Immunization Instructions

◆ **General questions and instructions**

Do you have a record of his/her immunizations?

Has he/she ever had a bad reaction to a vaccination?
Which vaccination?
What happened?

Does he/she have any allergies?

Does he/she have any illnesses?

Has he/she ever had a seizure?

Is there any possibility that she/you is pregnant?

Has he/she received immune globulin or other blood products (such as a transfusion) during the past several months?

Does your child or anyone at home have a weakened immune system; eg, by cancer, chemotherapy, treatment with steroids, or AIDS?

Instrucciones Para la Inmunización

◆ **Preguntas e instrucciones generales**

¿Tiene un registro de sus vacunas?

¿Ha tenido él/ella una mala reacción a alguna vacuna?
¿Qué vacuna?
¿Qué le pasó?

¿Tiene alergias?

¿Tiene alguna enfermedad?

¿Alguna vez ha tenido una convulsión?

¿Hay alguna posibilidad de que ella/usted este embarazada?

¿Ha recibido inmunoglobulina u otros productos sanguíneos (como transfusiones) en los últimos meses?

¿Tiene su niño/a o alguien en la casa un sistema inmune que este débil; por ejemplo, por cancer, quimioterapia, tratamiento con esteroides, o SIDA?

◆ **General questions and instructions (continued)**

As with any medicine, there are very small risks that serious problems, even death, could occur after getting a vaccine.

The risks from the vaccine are much smaller than the risks from the diseases if people stopped using the vaccine.

It is very common to get fever, fussiness, tenderness, and swelling from an immunization.

You can give him/her acetaminophen/cold compresses for this.

◆ **Preguntas e instrucciones generales (continuación)**

Como con cualquier otra medicina, existe el riesgo muy reducido de que, después de recibir la vacuna, pudieran ocurrir problemas serios incluyendo la muerte.

Los riesgos que presenta la vacuna son mucho menores que los riesgos de las enfermedades que resultarían si la gente dejara de vacunarse.

Es muy común tener fiebre, agitación, dolor e hinchazón por las vacunas.

Puede darle acetaminofen/ compresas frías para esto.

◆ **Diphtheria, tetanus, pertussis (DTP)**

Has your child ever had a seizure?

Some side effects are:

pain and redness at injection site

fever within 48 hours

tiredness, loss of appetite

allergic reaction

inflammation of the brain

seizure

"shock-collapse"

These risks are very low, and are higher for unvaccinated children.

◆ *Haemophilus Influenzae B:*

a bacteria called *Haemophilus* that can cause dangerous infections in children

Some side effects are:

pain and redness at the site of injection

fever

allergic reaction

◆ **Difteria, tétanos, tos convulsiva o ferina**

¿Ha tenido su niño/a convulsiones alguna vez?

Algunos efectos secundarios son:

dolor y enrojecimiento en el sitio de la inyección

fiebre en las siguientes cuarentiocho horas

cansancio, pérdida de apetito

reacción alérgica

inflamación del cerebro

una convulsión

choque o colapso

Estos riesgos son muy bajos, y son peor para niños no vacunados.

◆ *Haemophilus Influenza B:*

una bacteria llamada *Haemophilus* que puede causar infecciones peligrosas en niños

Algunos efectos secundarios son:

dolor y enrojecimiento en el sitio de la inyección

fiebre

reacción alérgica

- *Hepatitis A:* a virus that may infect the liver

  Some side effects are:

  pain and redness at the site of injection

  headache

  loss of appetite

  tiredness

- *Hepatitis B:* a virus that may infect the liver

  Some side effects are:

  pain and redness at the site of injection

  fever

- **Measles, mumps, rubella**

  Is your child allergic to eggs or neomycin?

  Does the child have a weakened immune system; eg, by cancer, chemotherapy, or treatment with steroids or AIDS?

  Is there any possibility that she/you is pregnant?

- *Hepatitis A:* un virus que puede infectar el hígado

  Éstos son algunos de los efectos colaterales:

  dolor y enrojecimiento donde se puso la inyecc

  dolor de cabeza

  pérdida del apetito

  cansansio

- *Hepatitis B:* un virus que puede infectar el hígado (hepatitis)

  Algunos efectos secundarios son:

  dolor y enrojecimiento en el sitio de la inyección

  fiebre

- **Sarampión, paperas, rubéola (sarampión alemán)**

  ¿Es su niño/a alérgico/a al huevo o al antibiótico neomicina?

  ¿Tiene su niño/a un sistema inmune que esté débil; por ejemplo por cáncer, quimioterapia, o tratamiento con esteroides o SIDA?

  ¿Hay alguna posibilidad de que ella/usted esté embarazada?

Some side effects are:

fever to 103° in
1 to 2 weeks

a rash

arthritis (transitory)
allergic reaction
seizure

◆ **Pneumococcal
infection:** may cause
serious infections
pneumonia and
meningitis

Some side effects are:

pain and redness at
the site of injection

fever
fussiness

◆ **Polio**

Does your child or
anyone at home have
a weakened immune
system; eg, by cancer,
chemotherapy, treatment
with steroids, or AIDS?

Side effects: paralysis
(very rare, less than 1
per million vaccines)

Algunos efectos
secundarios son:

fiebre hasta 103
(cientotres) grados
en una a dos semanas

una erupción/un
brote

artritis (transitoria)
reacción alérgica
convulsión

◆ **Infección por
neumococo:** puede
causar neumonía y
meningitis, dos
infecciones muy serias

Éstos son algunos de
los efectos colaterales:

dolor y enrojecimiento
donde se puso la
inyección

fiebre
irritabilidad

◆ **Polio**

¿Tiene su niño/a o
alguien en la casa un
sistema inmune que este
débil; por ejemplo por
cáncer, quimioterapia,
tratamiento con
esteroides, o SIDA?

Efectos secundarios:
parálisis (muy pocas
veces, menos que un
caso de polio por cada
millón de vacunas)

27

◆ **Varicella**

Has he/she/you ever had a serious allergic reaction to chickenpox vaccine, neomycin, or gelatin?

Is there any possibility that she/you is pregnant?

Does he/she/you or anyone at home have a weakened immune system; eg, by cancer, chemotherapy, radiation therapy, treatment with steroids, or AIDS?

Some side effects are:

pain and redness at injection site

fever

mild chickenpox rash

allergic reaction

seizure

◆ **Varicela**

¿Ha tenido alguna reacción alérgica a la vacuna contra varicela, al antibiótico neomicina, o a la gelatina?

¿Hay alguna posibilidad de que ella/usted esté embarazada?

¿Tiene él/ella/usted o alguien en la casa un sistema inmune que está débil, por ejemplo por cáncer, quimioterapia, terapia de rayos X, tratamiento con esteroides, o SIDA?

Algunos efectos secundarios son:

dolor y enrojecimiento en el sitio de la inyección

fiebre

erupción leve de varicela

reacción alérgica

un ataque o convulsión

Discharge Instructions	Instrucciones Para el Alta

1. Medication
2. General Instructions
3. Fever
4. Gastrointestinal
5. Respiratory
6. Neurology
7. Dermatology
8. Musculoskeletal Trauma

(Words often used in following section are provided here; for additional words, see pages 197-208.)

one	uno/a
two	dos
three	tres
four	cuatro
five	cinco
six	seis
as needed	como sea necesario

1. Medication

1. Medication	1. Medicación
Take _____ pills _____ times per day. (tablets, teaspoons, tablespoons, dropperfuls)	Tome _____ pastillas _____ veces al día (tabletas, cucharaditas, cucharadas, goteros)
Place _____ drops in	Póngale _____ gotas en
each ear	cada oído
each eye	cada ojo
right ear	el oído derecho
right eye	el ojo derecho
left ear	el oído izquierdo
left eye	el ojo izquierdo
_____ times per day.	_____ veces al día.

29

1. Medication (continued)

Place the ointment in
  each eye
  the right eye
  the left eye
  _____ times per day.

Apply the cream
(ointment)
  _____ times per day.

Take _____ puffs/
inhalations
  _____ times per day.

Place _____cc of _____
into _____ cc of
(normal saline) in the
nebulizer (machine).

Your child should
receive _____nebulizer
treatments per day.

Give your child the
medication only
when you feel
he/she needs it.

1. Medicación (continuación)

Póngale el ungüento
  en cada ojo
  el ojo derecho
  el ojo izquierdo
  _____ veces al día.

Póngale la crema
(el ungüento)
  _____ veces al día.

Tome _____
inhalaciones
  _____ veces al día.

Póngale _____ cc de
_____ en _____cc de
(agua salina) en el
nebulizador (maquina).

Su niño/a debe
recibir _____
tratamientos con
el nebulizador al día.

Dele a su niño/a la
medicina solamente
cuando usted crea
que él/ella la necesita.

2. General Instructions

Go to the nearest emergency department now.

Observe your child carefully.

Some danger signs are if your baby:
  becomes lethargic/tired
  cries a lot
  plays less
  does not eat well

If your child gets worse:
  Bring him/her to the emergency room. Return immediately.

Call the clinic if your child is not improving.

Return (tomorrow, in _____days, weeks, months).

I would like to see your child again in _____ (days, weeks, months, years).

Here is an appointment for _____.

2. Instrucciones Generales

Vaya al servicio de urgencias cercano ahora.

Observe a su niño/a con atención.

Son señas de peligro si su niño/a:
  se pone letárgico/a
  llora mucho
  juega menos
  no come bien

Si se empeora su niño/a:
  Traígalo/la a la sala de emergencias; Regresen inmediatamente.

Llame a la clínica si su niño/a no está mejorando.

Regresen (mañana; en _____ días, semanas, meses).

Quiero ver a su niño/a otra vez en _____ (días, semanas, meses, años).

Aquí tiene una cita para _____.

3. Fever

Take your child's temperature (every _____ hours, _____ times a day).

To take your child's temperature, place the thermometer in his/her (mouth, rectum, armpit) for 3 to 5 minutes.

Please call me (return to the clinic) if his/her temperature is greater than _____ degrees Celsius/Fahrenheit.

To help your child's fever go down, dress him/her in light clothing. You may also bathe him/her in lukewarm water for 15 to 20 minutes. Take him/her out if he/she begins to shiver.

Give your child lots of fluid to drink.

3. Fiebre

Tómele la temperatura (cada _____ horas, _____ veces al día).

Para tomar la temperatura, póngale el termómetro en su (boca, recto, axila) por tres a cinco minutos.

Llámeme (regresen a la clínica) si su temperatura es más de _____ grados Celsius/Fahrenheit.

Para bajar la temperatura, debe vestirle con ropa ligera. También puede bañarlo/la en agua tibia por quince a veinte minutos. Si comienza él/ella a tiritar, sáquelo/la del baño.

Déle a su niño/a mucho líquido para tomar.

4. Gastrointestinal

Try to give your child _____ (tablespoons, ounces, cups) of _____ (oral rehydration solution) every _____ hours for _____ days.

You can use a (spoon, dropper, syringe).

Give your child (regular formula, milk, juice) half diluted with water for _____ hours/days.

Do not give your child milk or dairy products for _____ days.

Foods which may help your child's diarrhea/constipation are:

Diarrhea

rice cereal

rice

potatoes (not fried)

noodles

crackers

toast

bananas

4. Gastrointestinal

Trate de darle a su niño/a _____ (cucharadas, onzas, tazas) de _____ (suero) cada _____ horas por_____ días.

Puede usar (una cuchara, un gotero, una jeringa).

Déle a su niño/a (fórmula, leche, jugo) diluido a la mitad con agua por _____ horas/días.

No le de leche o productos lácteos por _____ días.

Comidas que pueden mejorar la diarrea/el estreñamiento son:

Diarrea

cereal de arroz

arroz

papas (no fritas)

fideos

galletas saltinas

pan tostado

bananas

Constipation	**Estreñimiento**
fruit juices	jugos de fruta
apricot juice	jugo de durazno
apple juice	jugo de manzana
prune juice	jugo de pruna/ ciruela seca
bran cereal	cereal con fibra
bran muffins	panecillos (muffins) con fibra
whole wheat bread	pan integral
applesauce	puré de manzana

5. Respiratory

Some danger signs are:

- increased difficulty breathing
- pale or blue lip/skin color
- decreased eating or drinking
- problems taking the bottle
- faster breathing
- unusual drowsiness or fussiness

Place a humidifier in your child's bedroom.

5. Respiratorio

Señas de peligro son:

- más dificultad para respirar
- labios o piel de color pálido o azul
- disminución en lo que come o bebe
- problemas tomando la botella
- respiraciones más rápidas
- cansancio o irritabilidad

Ponga un humedificador en el dormitorio de su niño/a.

If your child has trouble breathing:	Si su niño/a tiene dificultad para respirar:
have him/her sit in the bathroom to breathe in the steam of a hot shower.	llévelo/la al cuarto de baño para respirar el vapor de una ducha caliente.
try taking him/her outside into the night air.	pruebe sacándolo/la al aire de la noche.

6. Neurology

Some danger signs are:

vomiting

dizziness

worsening headache

unsteadiness while walking

weakness of the arms or legs

abnormal sleepiness

confusion

difficulty speaking

If he/she shows any of these signs, call the clinic (bring him/her to the emergency department).

6. Neurológico

Algunas señas de peligro son:

vómitos

mareos

dolor de cabeza que empeora

inestabilidad cuando camina

debilidad en los brazos o piernas

cansancio más que lo normal

confusión

dificultad para hablar

Si muestra él/ella alguna de estas señas, llame a la clínica (traiga él/su al servicio de urgencias).

7. Dermatology

To decrease the itching, you may give your child a bath in lukewarm water (with _____).

You should soak the _____ in warm water for _____ minutes _____ times per day.

8. Musculoskeletal Trauma

Apply ice (a warm compress) for _____ minutes _____ times per day (before/after exercise).

He/she/you should rest (this, the _____) for _____ days.

You will need to use (crutches, an Ace bandage, a sling, a cast) for _____ (days, weeks).

He/she/you should elevate his/her/your _____ (hand, arm, foot, leg).

7. Dermatológico

Para qué no pique tanto, puede darle a su niño/a un baño con agua tibia (con _____).

Debe remojar el/la _____ en agua caliente por _____ minutos _____ veces al día.

8. Trauma Musculoesquelético

Aplique hielo (una compresa cálida) por _____ minutos _____ veces al día (antes/después del ejercicio).

Debe descansar (esto, el/la _____) por _____ días.

Vas a tener que usar (muletas, un vendaje "Ace," un cabestrillo, un yeso) por _____ (dias, semanas).

Debe elevar su _____ (mano, brazo, pie, pierna).

Stage Visit: Prenatal

History	Historia
◆ **Pregnancy**	◆ **Embarazo**
Have you had any problems with the pregnancy?	¿Ha tenido algún problema con el embarazo?
When is the baby due?	¿Cuándo debe nacer su bebe?
Have you been ill during your pregnancy? Diabetes? High blood pressure?	¿Ha tenido usted alguna enfermedad durante el embarazo? ¿Diabetes? ¿Presión alta?
Have you taken any medications? Alcohol? Smoke cigarettes? Use drugs?	¿Ha tomado usted algún medicamento? ¿Alcohol? ¿Fuma cigarrillos? ¿Usa drogas?
◆ **Family/social history**	◆ **Historia familiar/social**

(See pp. 12-18 for complete FH/SH.)

Are there any diseases that run in your family?	¿Hay alguna enfermedad en la familia?
Birth defects? Diabetes? Allergies? Asthma?	¿Defectos de nacimiento? ¿Diabetes? ¿Alergias? ¿Asma?
How old are you?	¿Cuántos años tiene usted?
Are you married, single, or with a partner?	¿Está casada, soltera, o convive?
Do you have other children? How old? Are they healthy?	¿Tiene más hijos? ¿De qué edades? ¿Están sanos?

◆ **Family/social history (continued)**

How many times have you been pregnant?

Have you had any miscarriages? Abortions?

Who lives at home with you?

Is the baby's father involved in the family?

Is there anyone to help you with the baby after the baby is born?

Where will your baby sleep?

Do you have a crib?

Do you work? What do you do?

Who will take care of the child while you work?

◆ **Nutrition**

Are you planning to breastfeed?

Will you be using formula?

◆ **Historia familiar/ social (continuación)**

¿Cuántas veces ha estado embarazada?

¿Ha tenido alguna pérdida? ¿Abortos?

¿Quién vive en casa con ustedes?

¿Está el padre del bebé involucrado con la familia?

¿Hay alguien que va a ayudarle con su bebé después de nacer?

¿Dónde va a dormir su bebe?

¿Tiene usted una cuna?

¿Usted trabaja? ¿Qué hace usted?

¿Quién va a cuidar al bebé cuándo usted trabaje?

◆ **Nutrición**

¿Piensa darle del pecho?

¿Va a darle fórmula?

◆ Circumcision

If you have a boy, do you want him to have a circumcision?

◆ Sleeping arrangements

Your baby should sleep on his/her back or side to reduce the small risk of SIDS.

Do not overheat your baby with blankets.

It is dangerous to sleep with the baby in your bed.

◆ Safety

Do you have a car seat for your baby? You need one to leave the hospital.

Do you have smoke detectors at home? You need them.

◆ Closing questions

Do you have any questions?

Congratulations!

◆ Circuncision

¿Si tuviese un niño, quisiera hacerle la circuncisión?

◆ Arreglos para dormir

Su bebé debe dormir boca arriba o de lado para reducir el pequeño riesgo del síndrome de muerte súbita, SIDS.

Evite sobrecalentar al bebé arropándolo más de la cuenta.

Es peligroso poner al bebé a dormir en la cama de usted.

◆ Seguridad

¿Tiene una silla para niños en el carro? La necesitan para salir del hospital.

¿Tienen detectores de humo en la casa? Los necesitan.

◆ Preguntas de despedida

¿Tiene algunas preguntas?

¡Felicitaciones!

Stage Visit: Newborn

History	Historia
◆ **Brief history**	◆ **Historia breve**
Congratulations!	¡Felicitaciones!
How are you doing?	¿Cómo está?
How are things going for you?	¿Cómo le va?
How was your delivery?	¿Cómo fue el parto?
How is your baby?	¿Cómo está su bebé?
Do you have any special concerns or questions?	¿Tiene usted alguna preocupación o pregunta en especial?
◆ **Pregnancy**	◆ **Embarazo**
Were there any problems with the pregnancy?	¿Hubo algún problema con el embarazo?
When was the baby due?	¿Cuándo debía nacer su bebé?
Were you ill during your pregnancy?	¿Tuvo usted alguna enfermedad durante el embarazo?
Diabetes? High blood pressure?	¿Diabetes? ¿Presión alta?
Did you take any medications? Alcohol? Smoke cigarettes? Use drugs?	¿Tomó usted algún medicamento? ¿Alcohol? ¿Fumó cigarrillos? ¿Usó drogas?

◆ Historia familiar/social
(See pp. 12-18 for complete FH/SH.)

Are there any diseases that run in your family?	¿Hay alguna enfermedad en la familia?
Birth defects? Diabetes? Allergies? Asthma?	¿Defectos de nacimiento? ¿Diabetes? ¿Alergias? ¿Asma?
How old are you?	¿Cuántos años tiene usted?
Are you married, single, or with a partner?	¿Está casada, soltera, o convive?
Do you have other children? How old? Are they healthy?	¿Tiene más hijos? ¿De qué edades? ¿Están sanos?
How many times have you been pregnant?	¿Cuántas veces ha estado embarazada?
Have you had any miscarriages? Abortions?	¿Ha tenido alguna pérdida? ¿Aborto?
Who lives at home with you?	¿Quién vive en casa con ustedes?
Is the baby's father involved in the family?	¿Está el padre del bebé involucrado con la familia?
Is there anyone to help you with the baby when you go home?	¿Hay alguien que va a ayudarle con su bebé cuando vuelva a casa?

41

◆ **Family/social history (continued)**

Do you work? What do you do?

Who will take care of the child while you work?

◆ **Historia familiar/social (continuación)**

¿Usted trabaja? ¿Qué hace usted?

¿Quién va a cuidar al bebé cuándo usted trabaje?

Physical Exam

height, weight, head circumference

maturity, jaundice, birth trauma

congenital anomalies

red reflex

femoral pulses

genitalia, descent of testes

hips, feet, spine

grasp, suck, walk, Moro reflex, muscle tone

Developmental Exam

parent-child interaction, feeding

startle, self-quieting, consolability

reaction to voice, fix and follow face

Intervention

♦ **Exam comments**

You have a beautiful baby.

He/she looks healthy and completely normal.

This is normal.

The rest of the umbilical cord will fall off in 1 to 2 weeks.

Call a doctor for excessive inflammation or bleeding.

Do not retract the foreskin of an uncircumcised baby.

A baby's breasts may be enlarged and leak milk.

Your baby may bleed a little from her vagina.

This is a normal effect of the mother's hormones, and will soon go away by itself.

Intervención

♦ **Comentarios del exámen**

Usted tiene un/a bebé muy lindo/a.

Él/ella parece sano/a y completamente normal.

Esto es normal.

El resto del cordón umbilical se caerá en una a dos semanas.

Llame al médico si se inflama o sangra demasiado.

No retraiga el prepucio si el niño no tiene circuncisión.

Los pechos de un bebé pueden ser grandes y producir leche.

Su bebé puede sangrar un poco por la vagina.

Eso es un efecto normal de las hormonas de la madre y desaparecerá por sí mismo dentro de poco.

◆ Feeding

Are you planning to breastfeed?

Have you started already?

Any problems or questions?

You may have only a little milk at first, but it will come.

Your baby should feed whenever he/she is hungry.

If your nipples become sore, you can help them by: breastfeeding for a shorter time but more often, or drying your nipples in the air or near a light bulb.

Breastfeeding does not prevent pregnancy.

Will you be using formula? What type?

A newborn can drink between 2 and 4 ounces.

◆ Alimentación

¿Piensa darle del pecho (alimento materno)?

¿Ya lo ha empezado?

¿Hay algún problema o pregunta?

Usted puede tener poca leche al comienzo, pero tendrá más.

Su bebé debe comer cada vez que tiene hambre.

Si le duelen los pezones, puede ayudarlos: dando el pecho menos tiempo pero con más frecuencia, o secando los pezones al aire o cerca un bombillo.

La lactancia materna no previene el embarazo.

¿Va a darle fórmula? ¿Qué tipo?

Un recién nacido puede beber entre dos y cuatro onzas.

◆ Basic functions

Babies sleep 2 to 4 hours at a time, 15 to 18 hours a day.

Some babies cry up to 2 to 3 hours a day.

His/her stools may be green, yellow, or brown.

After bowel movements, it is best to clean him/her with a moist towel.

You should bathe him/her no more than once a day.

◆ Mother

You should drink lots of liquids and get as much rest as possible.

Are you interested in birth control (family planning)?

Do you have a postnatal appointment with your OB/GYN?

◆ Funciones básicas

Los bebés duermen dos a cuatro horas a la vez, quince a dieciocho horas al día.

Algunos bebés lloran hasta dos a tres horas al día.

Su deposición puede ser de color verde, amarillo, o café.

Después de cada deposición, es mejor limpiarlo/a con una toalla mojada.

Debe bañarlo/a no más que una vez al día.

◆ Madre

Usted debe tomar mucho líquido y descansar lo más que pueda.

¿Quiere control de la natalidad (planificación familiar)?

¿Tiene usted una cita de postparto con su ginecólogo/a?

◆ **Safety**

Do you have a car seat for your baby?

It is very important always to use a car seat.

Do you have smoke detectors at home? You need them.

Be careful that your child doesn't fall from heights; for example, beds, cribs, and tables.

Your baby should sleep on his/her back or side to reduce the small risk of SIDS.

It is important to use a high-factor sunscreen (SPF 30 or more) on your child when he/she is outdoors.

◆ **Seguridad**

¿Tiene una silla para niños en el carro?

Es muy importante usar siempre una silla para niños en el carro.

¿Tienen detectores de humo en la casa? Los necesitan.

Tenga cuidado con lugares altos de donde pudiera él/ella caerse; por ejemplo, la cama, la cuna, y la mesa.

Su bebé debe dormir boca arriba o de lado para reducir el pequeño riesgo del síndrome de muerte súbita, SIDS.

Es importante aplicarle un aceite bronceador con protector solar de número alto (SPF treinta o mayor) cuando esté en el sol.

◆ Return instructions

Call the doctor if your baby:

> does not look well
>
> has a fever
>
> refuses to feed
>
> regurgitates or vomits often
>
> seems very irritable or sleepy

◆ Instrucciones de retorno

Llame al médico si su bebé:

> no se le ve bien
>
> tiene fiebre
>
> no quiere comer
>
> regurgita o vomita mucho
>
> está muy irritable o somnoliento

◆ Immunization & lab considerations
(See immunization schedule, Appendix.)

Vitamin/fluoride supplements if appropriate

I am going to give you vitamins and fluoride for his/her bones and teeth.

Voy a darle vitaminas y fluoruro para sus huesos y dientes.

Stage Visit: 2 to 4 weeks

History
◆ Chief complaint

What brings you in today?

Have you brought your baby for a routine checkup?

How is your baby?

Do you have any concerns or particular questions?

Since leaving the hospital, has your baby had any illness? Accident? Taken any medicine?

◆ Pregnancy

Were there any problems with the pregnancy?

Were you ill during your pregnancy?

Diabetes?
High blood pressure?

Did you take any medications? Alcohol? Smoke cigarettes? Use drugs?

Historia
◆ Molestia principal

¿Qué les trae por acá hoy?

¿Trae a su bebé para un chequeo de rutina?

¿Cómo está su bebé?

¿Tiene usted alguna preocupación o pregunta en especial?

¿Desde que salió del hospital, ha tenido su bebé alguna enfermedad? ¿Accidente? ¿Recibió alguna medicina?

◆ Embarazo

¿Hubo algún problema con el embarazo?

¿Tuvo usted alguna enfermedad durante el embarazo? ¿Diabetes? ¿Presión alta?

¿Tomó usted algún medicamento? ¿Alcohol? ¿Fumó cigarrillos? ¿Usó drogas?

◆ Delivery

When was your baby born? At which hospital?

What was the due date?

Did you deliver vaginally or by cesarean?

Were there any problems with the delivery?

Was the delivery spontaneous or induced?

Did the baby breathe right away?

Do you know the baby's Apgar scores?

How much did your baby weigh at birth?

Did he/she receive the Hepatitis B vaccine?

How many days did your baby spend in the hospital?

Was your baby sick while in the hospital?

◆ Parto

¿Cuándo nació su bebé? ¿En qué hospital?

¿Cuál era su fecha de parto?

¿Fue el parto vaginal o por operación cesárea?

¿Hubo algún problema con el parto?

¿Fue el parto espontáneo (natural) o provocado?

¿Respiró su bebé inmediatamente después de nacer?

¿Sabe los puntajes de Apgar que tuvo su bebé?

¿Cuánto pesó su bebé al nacer?

¿Recibió él/ella la vacuna contra la Hepatitis B?

¿Cuántos días pasó su bebé en el hospital?

¿Estuvo su bebé enfermo/a en el hospital?

◆ **Nutrition**

Are you breastfeeding?
How many times a day?

Are there any problems
with breastfeeding?
Questions?

Are you using formula?
What type?
How many ounces
a day?

How many ounces
at each feeding?
How frequently?

◆ **Behavior**

Does your baby
seem happy?

Are you enjoying
your baby?

For how long does
he/she sleep at
one time?

How many stools
per day?

How are they? Soft,
hard, watery?

Have you seen him/her
urinate? Is there a
good stream?

◆ **Nutrición**

¿Le da del pecho?
¿Cuántas veces al
día?

¿Tiene algún
problema con la
lactancia materna?
¿Preguntas?

¿Le da fórmula?
¿De qué tipo?
¿Cuántas onzas
al día?

¿Cuántas onzas
a la vez? ¿Con qué
frecuencia?

◆ **Comportamiento**

¿Le parece alegre
su bebé?

¿Disfruta usted a
su bebé?

¿Por cuánto tiempo
duerme él/ella a la
vez?

¿Cuántas veces
hace popó (evacua)
al día?

¿Cómo es la
evacuación? ¿Suave,
duro, aguado?

¿Lo/la ha visto
orinar? ¿Es fuerte
el chorro?

How many times per day does he/she wet his/her diaper?	¿Cuántos pañales moja al día?
Is your child crying too much?	¿Llora demasiado su bebé?

◆ **Family/social history**

◆ **Historia familiar/social**

Are there any diseases that run in your family? Diabetes? Cardiac defects? Tuberculosis? Asthma?	¿Hay alguna enfermedad en la familia? ¿Diabetes? ¿Defecto cardíaco? ¿Tuberculosis? ¿Asma?
How old are you?	¿Cuántos años tiene usted?
Are you married, single, or with a partner? Do you have other children? How old? Are they healthy?	¿Está casada, soltera, o convive? ¿Tiene más hijos? ¿De qué edades? ¿Están sanos?
How many times have you been pregnant?	¿Cuántas veces ha estado embarazada?
Have you had any miscarriages? Abortions?	¿Ha tenido alguna pérdida? ¿Aborto?
Who lives at home with you?	¿Quién vive en casa con ustedes?
Is the baby's father involved in the family?	¿Está el padre del bebé involucrado con la familia?

◆ **Family/social history (continued)**

Do you work?
What do you do?

Who takes care of the child while you work?

Do you have WIC?

Do you know how to apply for WIC?

Do you have Medicaid?
Health insurance?

◆ **Historia familiar/ social (continuación)**

¿Trabaja usted?
¿Qué hace?

¿Quién cuida al bebé cuándo usted trabaja?

¿Tienen WIC?

¿Sabe usted cómo solicitar WIC?

¿Tienen Medicaid?
¿Seguro médico?

Development

Can he/she see?

Does he/she react to sounds?

Can he/she lift her head off the bed?

Desarrollo

¿Cree que él/ella ve bien?

¿Reacciona él/ella al ruido?

¿Puede levantar la cabeza de la cama?

Physical Exam

hearing

height, weight, head circumference

congenital anomalies

red reflex, react to sound

grasp, suck, walk, Moro reflex

genitalia, hip click, tibial torsion, metatarsus adductus

Developmental Exam

Gross Motor: lift head off bed

Visual Motor: follows past midline

Language: may vocalize

Social: regards face

52

Intervention

◆ **Mother**

Are you still having vaginal bleeding? How many pads per day?

Are you having vaginal discharge? Does it smell bad?

Are you interested in birth control (family planning)?

Do you have a postnatal appointment with your OB/GYN?

◆ **Safety**

Do you have a car seat for your baby?

It is very important always to use a car seat.

Be careful that your child doesn't fall from heights; for example, beds, cribs, and tables.

Your baby should sleep on his/her back or side to reduce the small risk of SIDS.

Never leave the baby in direct sunlight because the skin may burn.

Intervención

◆ **Madre**

¿Sangra usted todavía de la vagina? ¿Cuántas toallas higiénicas usa al día?

¿Tiene flujo vaginal? ¿Huele mal?

¿Quiere control de la natalidad (planificación familiar)?

¿Tiene usted una cita de postparto con su ginecólogo/a?

◆ **Seguridad**

¿Tiene una silla para niños en el carro?

Es muy importante usar siempre una silla para niños en el carro.

Tenga cuidado con lugares altos de donde él/ella pudiera caerse; como por ejemplo, la cama, la cuna, y la mesa.

Su bebé debe dormir boca arriba o de lado para reducir el pequeño riesgo de síndrome de muerte súbita.

Nunca deje al bebé bajo la luz directa del sol porque la piel se le puede quemar.

◆ **Safety**

Are you concerned about violence in your home or neighborhood?

◆ **Seguridad**

¿Le preocupa la violencia en su casa o vecindario?

◆ **Immunization & lab considerations**

(Seee immunization schedule, Appendix.)

Vitamin/fluoride supplements if appropriate

I am going to give you vitamins and fluoride for his/her bones and teeth.

Voy a darle vitaminas y fluoruro para sus huesos y dientes.

Stage Visit: 2 months

History

◆ **Chief complaint**

What brings you in today?

Have you brought your baby for a routine checkup?

How is your baby?

Do you have any concerns or particular questions?

Since the last visit, has your baby had any illness? Accident? Taken any medicine?

◆ **Nutrition**

Are you breastfeeding? How many times a day?

Are there any problems with breastfeeding? Questions?

Are you using formula? What type? How many ounces per day?

How many ounces at each feeding? How frequently?

Do you have WIC?

Historia

◆ **Molestia principal**

¿Qué los trae por acá?

¿Trae a su bebé para un chequeo de rutina?

¿Cómo está su bebé?

¿Tiene usted alguna preocupación o pregunta en especial?

¿Desde la ultima visita, ha tenido su bebé alguna enfermedad? ¿Accidente? ¿Recibió alguna medicina?

◆ **Nutrición**

¿Le da usted el pecho? ¿Cuántas veces al día?

¿Hay algún problema con la lactancia materna? ¿Preguntas?

¿Le da fórmula? ¿De qué tipo? ¿Cuántas onzas al día?

¿Cuántas onzas a la vez? ¿Con qué frecuencia?

¿Tienen WIC?

Behavior

Does your baby seem happy?

Are you enjoying your baby?

For how long does he/she sleep at one time?

How many stools per day?
What are they like?
Soft, hard, watery?

Does your baby cry too much?

Development

What is he/she able to do now?

Can your baby:

follow you with his/her eyes?

react to sounds?

lift his/her head off the bed?

coo?

smile at you?

Comportamiento

¿Le parece alegre su bebé?

¿Goza usted a su bebé?

¿Por cuánto tiempo duerme él/ella a la vez?

¿Cuántas veces evacua (hace popó) al día? ¿Cómo son?
¿Suave, duro, aguado?

¿Llora demasiado su bebé?

Desarrollo

¿Qué puede hacer él/ella ahora?

¿Puede su bebé:

seguirle con sus ojos?

reaccionar a ruidos?

levantar la cabeza de la cama?

hacer "agu"?

sonreirse con usted?

Physical Exam	Developmental Exam
height, weight head circumference	Gross Motor: head up to 45°, may steady head
congenital anomalies	Visual Motor: follows past midline, relaxed fists
red reflex, react to sound	Language: coo
hip click, genitalia	Social: smile responsively
grasp, suck, Moro reflex	

Intervention

◆ **Mother**

Are you interested in birth control (family planning)?

◆ **Nutrition**

Do not give honey or solid foods.

◆ **Safety**

Do you have a car seat for your baby?

It is very important always to use a car seat.

He/she can now move and reach more easily.

Intervención

◆ **Madre**

¿Quiere control de la natalidad (planificación familiar)?

◆ **Nutrición**

No le dé miel o comida sólida.

◆ **Seguridad**

¿Tiene una silla para niños en el carro?

Es muy importante usar siempre una silla para niños en el carro.

Él/ella empieza a moverse y agarrar cosas.

◆ Safety (continued)

Careful that he/she:

- does not fall
- does not grab anything dangerous
- does not put small objects in mouth

Your baby should sleep on his/her back or side to reduce the small risk of SIDS.

You should use sunscreen to protect your baby's skin.

It is important to use a high-factor sunscreen (SPF 30 or more) on your child when he/she is outdoors.

◆ Seguridad (continuación)

Tenga cuidado que él/ella:

- no se caiga
- no agarre cosas peligrosas
- no lleve cosas pequeñas a la boca

Su bebé debe dormir boca arriba o de lado para reducir el pequeño riesgo de síndrome de muerte súbita.

Debe usar bloqueadores para proteger la piel de su bebé del sol.

Es importante aplicarle un aceite bronceador con protector solar de número alto (SPF treinta o mayor) cuando esté en el sol.

◆ Immunization & lab considerations
(See immunization schedule, Appendix.)

Hgb/Hct if indicated.

Stage Visit: 4 months

History

◆ **Chief complaint**

What brings you in today?

Have you brought your baby for a routine checkup?

How is your baby?

Do you have any concerns?

Since the last visit, has your baby had any illness? Accident? Taken any medicine?

◆ **Nutrition**

Are you breastfeeding? How many times a day?

Are you using formula? What type? How many ounces per day?

How many ounces at each feeding? How frequently?

Do you have WIC?

Historia

◆ **Molestia principal**

¿Qué los trae por acá?

¿Trae a su bebé para un chequeo de rutina?

¿Cómo está su bebé?

¿Tiene usted alguna preocupación o pregunta en especial?

¿Desde la última visita, ha tenido su bebé alguna enfermedad? ¿Accidente? ¿Recibió alguna medicina?

◆ **Nutrición**

¿Le da usted el pecho? ¿Cuántas veces al día?

¿Le da fórmula? ¿De qué tipo? ¿Cuántas onzas al día?

¿Cuántas onzas a la vez? ¿Con qué frecuencia?

¿Tienen WIC?

◆ **Behavior**

Does your baby seem happy?

Are you enjoying your baby?

For how long does he/she sleep at one time?

How many stools/day? What are they like? Soft, hard, watery?

◆ **Comportamiento**

¿Le parece alegre su bebé?

¿Disfruta usted a su bebé?

¿Por cuánto tiempo duerme él/ella a la vez?

¿Cuántas veces evacua al día? ¿Cómo son? ¿Suave, duro, aguado?

Development

What is he/she able to do now?

Can your baby:

lift his/her head and shoulders off the bed?

sit up with your help?

roll over?

reach for objects?

hold a toy in hand?

smile at you?

laugh or make any other noises?

Desarrollo

¿Qué puede hacer él/ella ahora?

¿Puede su bebé:

levantar la cabeza y los hombros de la cama?

estarse sentado/a con su ayuda?

darse vuelta?

estirar la mano para alcanzar objetos?

agarrar (aguantar) un juguete en la mano?

sonreirle?

reírse o hacer otro ruido?

60

Physical Exam

hearing

height, weight, head circumference

strabismus

hip click

Developmental Exam

Gross Motor: roll over with or without head lag, grasp toy, sit, bear weight on legs

Visual Motor: follow 180°, reach, responds to sound

Language: coo, laugh

Social: look around, anticipate feeding, vocalize responsively

Intervention
◆ **Instructions**

Your child should begin trying solid foods.

Start foods one at a time, no more than one every 2 or 3 days.

Some good foods to begin with are: rice cereal, bananas, applesauce.

Do not give honey or corn syrup.

Intervención
◆ **Instrucciones**

Su bebé debe empezar con un poco de comida sólida.

No empiece con más de un nuevo tipo de comida cada dos o tres días.

Son buenas comidas para empezar: el cereal de arroz, la banana, el puré de manzana.

No le dé miel ni almíbar de maíz.

◆ **Safety**

Make sure you use a car seat.

He/she can now move and reach more easily.

Careful that he/she:

does not fall
does not grab anything dangerous
does not put small objects in mouth

It is important to use a high-factor sunscreen (SPF 30 or more) on your child when he/she is outdoors.

Your baby should sleep on his/her back or side to reduce the small risk of SIDS.

Are you concerned about violence in your home or neighborhood?

◆ **Seguridad**

Asegúrese de usar una silla para niños en el carro.

Él/ella puede moverse y agarrar cosas.

Tenga cuidado que él/ella:

no se caiga
no agarre cosas peligrosas

no se lleve cosas pequeñas a la boca

Es importante aplicarle un aceite bronceador con protector solar de número alto (SPF treinta o mayor) cuando esté en el sol.

El bebé debe dormir boca arriba o de lado para reducir el pequeño riesgo del síndrome de muerte súbita, SIDS.

¿Le preocupa la violencia en su casa o vecindario?

◆ **Immunization & lab considerations**
   (See immunization schedule, Appendix.)
Hgb/Hct if indicated.

Stage Visit: 6 months

History

◆ **Chief complaint**

What brings you in today?

Have you brought your baby for a routine checkup?

How is your baby?

Do you have any concerns or particular questions?

Since the last visit, has your baby had any illness? Accident? Taken any medicine?

◆ **Nutrition**

Is your baby feeding well?

Are you breastfeeding? How many times a day?

Are you using formula? What type?

Is he/she eating solid foods? What kinds? How much?

Historia

◆ **Molestia principal**

¿Qué los trae por acá?

¿Trae a su bebé para un chequeo de rutina?

¿Cómo está su bebé?

¿Tiene usted alguna preocupación o pregunta en especial?

¿Desde la última visita, ha tenido su bebé alguna enfermedad? ¿Accidente? ¿Recibió alguna medicina?

◆ **Nutrición**

¿Come bien su bebé?

¿Le da usted el pecho? ¿Cuántas veces al día?

¿Le da fórmula? ¿De qué tipo?

¿Come él/ella comida sólida? ¿Cuáles? ¿Cuánto?

Behavior

Does your baby seem happy?

Are you enjoying your baby?

What do you do together?

For how long does he/she sleep at one time?

How many stools per day? What are they like? Soft, hard, watery?

Development

What is he/she able to do now?

Can your baby:

roll over?

sit up?

reach for objects?

eat with his/her fingers?

babble?

Comportamiento

¿Le parece alegre su bebé?

¿Disfruta usted a su bebé?

¿Qué cosas hacen ustedes juntos?

¿Cuánto tiempo duerme él/ella a la vez?

¿Cuántas veces evacua (hace popó) al día? ¿Cómo son? ¿Suave, duro, aguado?

Desarrollo

¿Qué puede hacer él/ella ahora?

¿Puede su bebé:

darse la vuelta?

estar sentado/a?

estirar la mano para alcanzar objetos?

comer con los dedos?

balbucear?

Physical Exam	**Developmental Exam**
height, weight, head circumference	Gross Motor: sit well, no head lag
strabismus	Visual Motor: raking
grasp, transfer	Language: babble
hip click	Social: eat finger foods
teeth (5 to 8 mos)	

Intervention
◆ Instructions

Continue breastfeeding or formula until 1 year old.

You can start giving fresh fruits and cooked vegetables.

Introduce only one new food every 2 to 3 days.

Intervención
◆ Instrucciones

Siga dándole el pecho o fórmula hasta el año.

Puede empezar a darle frutas frescas y verduras cocidas.

Dele solamente un nuevo tipo de comida cada dos o tres días.

◆ **Safety**

Be careful about him/her:

> falling (eg, down stairs)
>
> reaching for dangerous objects
>
> putting small things in mouth

You should use:

> car seats
>
> smoke detectors in the home
>
> locks for cabinets and windows
>
> outlet covers
>
> stairway gates
>
> sun protection

Be careful about the hot water temperature.

Reduce to 120° to prevent accidental burns.

◆ **Seguridad**

Tenga cuidado que el niño puede:

> caerse (por ejemplo, por la escalera)
>
> agarrar cosas peligrosas
>
> llevarse cosas pequeñas a la boca

Debe usar:

> una silla para niños en el carro
>
> detectores de humo en la casa
>
> seguros para armarios y ventanas
>
> cubiertas para los toma corrientes
>
> barreras para las escaleras
>
> protección contra el sol

Debe tener cuidado con la temperatura del agua caliente.

Rebájela a 120 (ciento veinte) grados para prevenir quemaduras.

Caution with pots on the stove. Turn handles so that your child cannot reach them.

Tenga cuidado con las ollas encima de la estufa. Voltée los agarraderos para que su niño/a no los alcance.

Place medications and chemicals out of reach.

Ponga medicinas y químicos lejos de su alcance.

In case of poisoning, call the Poison Control Center at #_____.

En caso de envenenamiento, llame al Poison Control Center (Centro Contra Envenenamiento): #_____.

It is important to use a high-factor sunscreen (SPF 30 or more) on your child when he/she is outdoors.

Es importante aplicarle un aceite bronceador con protector solar de número alto (SPF treinta o mayor) cuando esté en el sol.

Your baby should sleep on his/her back or side to reduce the small risk of SIDS.

El bebé debe dormir boca arriba o de lado para reducir el pequeño riesgo del síndrome de muerte súbita, SIDS.

♦ **Immunization & lab considerations**
    (See immunization schedule, Appendix.)

Stage Visit: 9 months

History

- **Chief complaint**

  What brings you in today?

  Have you brought your baby for a routine checkup?

  How is your baby?

  Do you have any concerns or particular questions?

  Since the last visit, has your baby had any illness? Accident? Taken any medicine?

- **Nutrition**

  Is your baby feeding well?

  Are you breastfeeding? How many times a day?

  Are you using formula? What type?

  Is he/she eating solid foods? What kinds? How much?

  Offer liquids in a cup.

Historia

- **Molestia principal**

  ¿Qué los trae por acá?

  ¿Trae a su bebé para un chequeo de rutina?

  ¿Cómo está su bebé?

  ¿Tiene usted alguna preocupación o pregunta en especial?

  ¿Desde la última visita, ha tenido su bebé alguna enfermedad? ¿Accidente? ¿Recibió alguna medicina?

- **Nutrición**

  ¿Come bien su bebé?

  ¿Le da usted el pecho? ¿Cuántas veces al día?

  ¿Le da fórmula? ¿De qué tipo?

  ¿Come él/ella comida sólida? ¿Cuáles? ¿Cuánto?

  Ofrezca las bebidas en un vaso.

◆ Behavior

Does your baby seem happy?

Are you enjoying your baby?

What do you do together?

Does he/she sleep through the night?

How many stools per day?
What are they like?
Soft, hard, watery?

Development

What is he/she able to do now?

Can your baby:

  sit well?

  crawl?

  stand holding on?

  eat with his/her fingers?

  babble?

  say any words?

  understand "no"?

  understand his/her name?

How does your baby react to strangers?

◆ Comportamiento

¿Le parece alegre su bebé?

¿Disfruta usted a su bebé?

¿Qué cosas hacen ustedes juntos?

¿Duerme toda la noche?

¿Cuántas veces hace popó al día?
¿Cómo son?
¿Suave, duro, aguado?

Desarrollo

¿Qué puede hacer él/ella ahora?

¿Puede su bebé:

  quedarse bien sentado/a?

  gatear?

  estar parado/a agarrándose de cosas?

  comer con los dedos?

  balbucear?

  decir alguna palabra?

  comprender "no"?

  entender su nombre?

¿Como reacciona su bebé frente a extraños?

Physical Exam

hearing

height, weight, head circumference

strabismus

hip click

teeth (5 to 8 mos)

Developmental Exam

Gross Motor: crawl, stand holding on

Visual Motor: pincer grasp, bang objects

Language: Babble, non-specific dada/mama

Social: bye-bye, pat-a-cake, show wants

Intervention
◆ **Instructions**

Start brushing his/her teeth.

Your child should begin eating normal food in small quantities.

Continue breastfeeding or formula until 1 year old.

Be careful with foods he/she can choke on.

Do not give:
peanuts, raisins, whole beans
large pieces of hot dog
raw vegetables, large pieces of fruit

Intervención
◆ **Instrucciones**

Empiece a cepillar sus dientes.

Su niño/a debe comer comida normal en cantidades pequeñas.

Siga dándole de mamar o fórmula hasta la edad de un año.

Cuidado con las comidas con las que pueda atragantarse.

No le dé:
maníes, pasas, frijoles enteros
pedazos grandes de hot dog (salchicha)
verduras crudas, pedazos grandes de fruta

70

◆ Safety

Be careful about him/her:

 falling (eg, down stairs)

 reaching for dangerous objects

 putting small objects in the mouth

You should use:

 car seats

 smoke detectors in the home

 locks for cabinets and windows

 outlet covers

 stairway gates

 sun protection

Be careful about the hot water temperature. Reduce to 120° to prevent accidental burns.

Your baby should sleep on his/her back or side to reduce the small risk of SIDS.

◆ Seguridad

Tenga cuidado que el niño puede:

 caerse (por ejemplo, por la escalera)

 agarrar cosas peligrosas

 llevarse cosas pequeñas a la boca

Debe usar:

 una silla para niños en el carro

 detectores de humo en la casa

 seguros para armarios y ventanas

 cobertores para los toma corrientes

 barreras para las escaleras

 protección contra el sol

Tenga cuidado con la temperatura del agua caliente. Rebájela a 120 (ciento veinte) grados para prevenir quemaduras accidentales.

Su bebé debe dormir boca arriba o de lado para reducir el pequeño riesgo de síndrome de muerte súbita, SIDS.

◆ **Safety
(continued)**

Are you concerned about violence in your home or neighborhood?

Caution with pots on the stove. Turn handles so that your child cannot reach them.

Place medications and chemicals out of reach.

In case of poisoning, call the Poison Control Center at #_____.

It is important to use a high-factor sunscreen (SPF 30 or more) on your child when he/she is outdoors.

◆ **Seguridad
(continuación)**

¿Le preocupa la violencia en su casa o vecindario?

Tenga cuidado con las ollas encima de la estufa. Voltee los agarraderos para que su niño/a no los alcance.

Ponga medicinas y químicos lejos de su alcance.

En caso de envenenamiento, llame al Poison Control Center (Centro Contra Envenenamiento): #_____.

Es importante aplicarle un aceite bronceador con protector solar de número alto (SPF treinta o mayor) cuando esté en el sol.

◆ **Immunization & lab considerations**
   (See immunization schedule, Appendix.)

Hgb/Hct (6 to 12 mos)
Pb if indicated
PPD if indicated

Stage Visit: 12 months

History

◆ **Chief complaint**

What brings you in today?

Have you brought your child for a routine checkup?

How is your child?

Do you have any concerns or particular questions?

Since the last visit, has your child had any illness? Accident? Taken any medicine?

◆ **Nutrition**

Is your child feeding well?

Are you still breastfeeding? How many times a day?

Are you still using formula? What type?

Is he/she eating solid foods? What kinds? How much?

Historia

◆ **Molestia principal**

¿Qué los trae por acá?

¿Trae a su niño/a para un chequeo de rutina?

¿Cómo está su niño/a?

¿Tiene usted alguna preocupación o pregunta en especial?

¿Desde la última visita, ha tenido su niño/a alguna enfermedad? ¿Accidente? ¿Recibió alguna medicina?

◆ **Nutrición**

¿Come bien su niño/a?

¿Le da usted el pecho todavía? ¿Cuántas veces al día?

¿Le da fórmula todavía? ¿De qué tipo?

¿Come él/ella comida sólida? ¿Cuáles? ¿Cuánto?

◆ **Behavior**

Does your child seem happy?

Are you enjoying your child?

What do you do together?

Does he/she sleep well?

How many stools per day?
What are they like?
Soft, hard, watery?

Development

What is he/she able to do now?

Can your child:
 walk holding on?

 walk?

 eat with his/her fingers?

 play peek-a-boo?

 say any words?

 understand "no"?

 understand his/her name?

◆ **Comportamiento**

¿Le parece alegre su niño/a?

¿Disfruta usted a su niño/a?

¿Qué cosas hacen ustedes juntos?

¿Duerme bien?

¿Cuántas veces hace popó al día?
¿Cómo son?
¿Suave, duro, aguado?

Desarrollo

¿Qué puede hacer él/ella ahora?

¿Puede su niño/a:
 andar agarrándose de cosas?

 caminar?

 comer con los dedos?

 jugar a esconderse?

 decir alguna palabra?

 comprender "no"?

 entender su nombre?

Physical Exam	Developmental Exam
height, weight, head circumference	Gross Motor: stand alone, walk, cruise
strabismus	Visual Motor: throw, drink from cup
vision, hearing	Language: 1 to 2 words
hips, gait	Social: imitate, play ball
teeth	

Intervention

◆ **Instructions**

Your child should be eating normal food.

He/she should start using a cup.

Be careful with foods he/she can choke on.

Do not give:
  peanuts, raisins, whole beans
  large pieces of hot dog

  raw vegetables, large pieces of fruit

You should brush his/her teeth with just a little toothpaste.

Intervención

◆ **Instrucciones**

Su niño/a debe comer comida normal.

Debe empezar a usar un vaso.

Tenga cuidado con las comidas con las que pueda atragantarse.

No le dé:
  maníes, pasas, frijoles enteros
  pedazos grandes de hot dog (salchicha)
  verduras crudas, pedazos grandes de fruta

Debe cepillar sus dientes con un poquito de pasta dental.

75

◆ **Instructions (continued)**

Talk with your baby frequently to help him/her learn to speak.

◆ **Safety**

Be careful about him/her:

falling (eg, down stairs)

reaching for dangerous objects

putting small objects in mouth

You should use:

car seats

smoke detectors in the home

locks for cabinets and windows

outlet covers

stairway gates

sun protection

◆ **Instrucciones (continuación)**

Hable mucho con su niño/a para ayudarle a aprender a hablar.

◆ **Seguridad**

Debe tener cuidado que el niño puede:

caerse (por ejemplo, por la escalera)

agarrar cosas peligrosas

llevarse cosas pequeñas a la boca

Debe usar:

una silla para niños en el carro

detectores de humo en la casa

seguros para armarios y ventanas

cubiertas para los toma corrientes

barreras para las escaleras

protección contra el sol

Be careful about
the hot water
temperature.
Reduce to 120° to
prevent accidental
burns.

Caution with pots on the
stove. Turn handles so
that your child cannot
reach them.

Place medications and
chemicals out of reach.

In case of poisoning,
call the Poison Control
Center at #_____.

Do you have any guns
in your home? If you
need to keep a gun in
your house, keep the
gun unloaded and
locked up. Store the
ammunition in a
different place away
from the gun.

Tenga cuidado con
la temperatura del
agua caliente.
Rebájela a 120 (ciento
veinte) grados para
prevenir quemaduras.

Tenga cuidado con
los ollas encima de
la estufa. Voltee los
agarraderos para
que su niño/a no los
alcance.

Ponga medicinas y
químicos lejos de
su alcance.

En caso de
envenenamiento,
llame al Poison
Control Center
(Centro Contra
Envenenamiento):
#_____.

¿Tiene armas en su
casa? Si usted
necesitara tener un
arma (de fuego) en la
casa, manténgala
descargada, en un
lugar seguro y bajo
llave. Mantenga las
municiones en un lugar
diferente a donde
guarda el arma.

◆ **Safety
(continued)**

It is important to use a high-factor sunscreen (SPF 30 or more) on your child when he/she is outdoors.

Your baby should sleep on his/her back or side to reduce the small risk of SIDS.

Are you concerned about violence in your home or neighborhood?

◆ **Seguridad
(continuación)**

Es importante aplicarle un aceite bronceador con protector solar de número alto (SPF treinta o mayor) cuando esté en el sol.

El bebé debe dormir boca arriba o de lado para reducir el pequeno riesgo de síndrome de muerte súbita, SIDS.

¿Le preocupa la violencia en su casa o vecindario?

◆ **immunization & lab considerations**
   (See immunization schedule, Appendix.)

Hgb/Hct (6 to 12 mos)
Pb if indicated
PPD if indicated

Stage Visit: 15 months

History	**Historia**
◆ **Chief complaint**	◆ **Molestia principal**
What brings you in today?	¿Qué les trae por acá?
Have you brought your child for a routine checkup?	¿Trae a su niño/a para un chequeo de rutina?
How is your child?	¿Cómo está su niño/a?
Do you have any concerns or particular questions?	¿Tiene usted alguna preocupación o pregunta en especial?
Since the last visit, has your child had any illness? Accident? Taken any medicine?	¿Desde la última visita, ha tenido su niño/a alguna enfermedad? ¿Accidente? ¿Recibió alguna medicina?
◆ **Nutrition**	◆ **Nutrición**
Is your child eating well?	¿Come bien su niño/a?
Are you still breastfeeding? How many times a day?	¿Le da usted el pecho todavía? ¿Cuántas veces al día?
What does he/she eat? How much? What does he/she like most?	¿Qué come él/ella? ¿Cuánto? ¿Qué es lo que más le gusta?

◆ **Behavior**	◆ **Comportamiento**
Does your child seem happy?	¿Le parece alegre su niño/a?
Are you enjoying your child?	¿Disfruta usted a su niño/a?
What do you do together?	¿Qué cosas hacen ustedes juntos?
Does he/she sleep well?	¿Duerme bien?
How many stools per day?	¿Cuántas veces hace popó al día?
What are they like?	¿Cómo son?
Soft, hard, watery?	¿Suave, duro, aguado?

Development / Desarrollo

What is he/she able to do now?	¿Qué puede hacer él/ella ahora?
Can your child:	¿Puede su niño/a:
walk?	andar?
crawl upstairs?	subir gradas ó escalones gateando?
eat with his/her fingers?	comer con los dedos?
use a cup?	tomar de un vaso?
scribble?	hacer garabatos?
say any words?	decir alguna palabra?
imitate what you do?	imitar lo que hace usted?

Physical Exam	**Developmental Exam**
height, weight, head circumference	Gross Motor: walk well, crawl upstairs, +/- run
strabismus	Visual Motor: scribble, drink from cup
vision, hearing	Language: 3 to 6 words
teeth	Social: imitate, play ball
gait	
hernias	

Intervention
◆ **Instructions**

Your child should be eating normal food.

Be careful with foods he/she can choke on.

Do not give:
  peanuts, raisins, whole beans

  large pieces of hot dog

  raw vegetables, large pieces of fruit

You should brush his/her teeth with just a little toothpaste.

Talk with your baby frequently to help him/her learn to speak.

He/she should have a regular bedtime.

Intervención
◆ **Instrucciones**

Su niño/a debe comer comida normal.

Tenga cuidado con las comidas con las que pueda atragantarse.

No le dé:
  maníes, pasas, frijoles enteros

  pedazos grandes de hot dog (salchicha)

  verduras crudas, pedazos grandes de fruta

Debe cepillar sus dientes con un poquito de pasta dental.

Hable mucho con su niño/a para ayudarle a aprender a hablar.

Su niño/a debe tener una hora fija para acostarse.

◆ **Instructions (continued)**

He/she should not watch too much television — better to play and read with him/her.

◆ **Safety**

You should use:
car seats

smoke detectors in the home
locks for cabinets and windows
outlet covers

stairway gates

sun protection

Be careful about the hot water temperature. Reduce to 120° to prevent accidental burns.

Caution with pots on the stove. Turn handles so that your child cannot reach them.

Are you concerned about violence in your home or neighborhood?

◆ **Instrucciones (continuación)**

No le permita ver mucha televisión — es mejor jugar y leer con él/ella.

◆ **Seguridad**

Debe usar:
una silla para niños en el carro
detectores de humo en la casa
seguros para armarios y ventanas
cubiertas para los toma corrientes
barreras para las escaleras
protección contra el sol

Tenga cuidado con la temperatura del agua caliente. Rebájela a 120 (ciento veinte) grados para prevenir quemaduras.

Tenga cuidado con las ollas encima de la estufa. Voltee los agarraderos para que su niño/a no los alcance.

¿Le preocupa la violencia en su casa o vecindario?

Place medications and chemicals out of reach.

Ponga medicinas y químicos lejos de su alcance.

In case of poisoning, call the Poison Control Center at #_____.

En caso de envenenamiento, llame al Poison Control Center (Centro Contra Envenenamiento): #_____.

Do you have any guns in your home? If you need to keep a gun in your house, keep the gun unloaded and locked up. Store the ammunition in a different place away from the gun.

¿Tiene armas en su casa? Si usted necesitara tener un arma (de fuego) en la casa, manténgala descargada, en un lugar seguro y bajo llave. Mantenga las municiones en un lugar diferente a donde guarda el arma.

Never leave your child alone near water — a bathtub, toilet, wells, swimming pool, lake, or ocean.

Nunca deje a su niño sin supervisión cerca del agua, como por ejemplo la bañera, el inodoro o excusado, pozos, piscinas, lagos, u océano.

It is important to use a high-factor sunscreen (SPF 30 or more) on your child when he/she is outdoors.

Es importante aplicarle un aceite bronceador con protector solar de numero alto (SPF treinta o mayor) cuando esté en el sol.

◆ **Immunization & lab considerations**
(See immunization schedule, Appendix.)

Pb if indicated
PPD if indicated

Hemoglobin or hematocrit if child is at risk

Stage Visit: 18 months

History	Historia

History

◆ **Chief complaint**

What brings you in today?

Have you brought your child for a routine checkup?

How is your child?

Do you have any concerns or particular questions?

Since the last visit, has your child had any illness? Accident? Taken any medicine?

◆ **Nutrition**

Is your child eating well?

Are you still breastfeeding? How many times a day?

What does he/she eat? How much? What does he/she like most?

Historia

◆ **Molestia principal**

¿Qué los trae por acá?

¿Trae a su niño/a para un chequeo de rutina?

¿Cómo está su niño/a?

¿Tiene usted alguna preocupación o pregunta en especial?

¿Desde la última visita, ha tenido su niño/a alguna enfermedad? ¿Accidente? ¿Recibió alguna medicina?

◆ **Nutrición**

¿Come bien su niño/a?

¿Le da usted el pecho todavía? ¿Cuántas veces al día?

¿Qué come él/ella? ¿Cuánto? ¿Qué es lo que más le gusta?

Behavior	Comportamiento
Does your child seem happy?	¿Le parece alegre su niño/a?
Are you enjoying your child?	¿Disfruta usted a su niño/a?
What do you do together?	¿Qué cosas hacen ustedes juntos?
Does he/she sleep well?	¿Duerme bien?
How many stools/day? What are they like? Soft, hard, watery?	¿Cuántas veces evacua al día? o ¿Cóm son? ¿Suave, duro, aguado?

Development	Desarrollo
What is he/she able to do now?	¿Qué puede hacer él/ella ahora?
Can your child:	¿Puede su niño/a:
walk upstairs?	subir gradas ó escalones andando?
run?	correr?
kick a ball?	patear un balón?
use a spoon?	comer con una cuchara?
remove some clothing?	quitarse la ropa?
turn pages of a book?	voltear las páginas de un libro?
say words?	decir palabras?

Physical Exam	Developmental Exam
height, weight, head circumference	Gross Motor: walk upstairs, run, kick ball
strabismus	Visual Motor: use spoon, crude page turning
vision, hearing	
teeth	Language: 6 + words
gait	Social: remove clothing
hernia	

Intervention

◆ **Instructions**

Your child should be eating normal food.

Be careful with foods he/she can choke on.

Do not give:
  peanuts, raisins, whole beans
  large pieces of hot dog

  raw vegetables, large pieces of fruit

You should brush his/her teeth with just a little toothpaste.

Talk to your baby frequently to help him/her learn to speak.

Intervención

◆ **Instrucciones**

Su niño/a debe comer comida normal.

Tenga cuidado con las comidas con las que pueda atragantarse.

No le dé:
  maníes, pasas, frijoles enteros
  pedazos grandes de hot dog (salchicha)
  verduras crudas, pedazos grandes de fruta

Debe cepillar sus dientes con un poquito de pasta dental.

Hable mucho con su niño/a para ayudarle a aprender a hablar.

He/she should have
a regular bedtime.

He/she should not watch
too much television —
it's better to play and
read with him/her.

◆ **Safety**

You should use:

car seats

smoke detectors
in the home

locks for cabinets
and windows

outlet covers

stairway gates

sun protection

Be careful about
the hot water
temperature.
Reduce to 120° to
prevent accidental
burns.

Su niño/a debe tener
una hora fija para
acostarse.

No le permita ver
mucha televisión —
es mejor jugar y
leer con él/ella.

◆ **Seguridad**

Debe usar:

una silla para
niños en el carro

detectores de
humo en la casa

seguros para
armarios y
ventanas

cubiertas para
los toma corrientes

barreras para
las escaleras

protección contra
el sol

Tenga cuidado
con la temperatura
del agua caliente.
Rebájela a 120 (ciento
veinte) grados para
prevenir quemaduras.

◆ **Safety (continued)**

Caution with pots on the stove. Turn handles so that your child cannot reach them.

Place medications and chemicals out of reach.

In case of poisoning, call the Poison Control Center at #_____.

Do you have any guns in your home? If you need to keep a gun in your house, keep the gun unloaded and locked up. Store the ammunition in a different place away from the gun.

Never leave your child alone near water — like a bathtub, toilet, wells, swimming pool, lake, or ocean.

◆ **Seguridad (continuación)**

Tenga cuidado con las ollas encima de la estufa. Voltee los agarraderos para que su niño/a no los alcance.

Ponga medicinas y químicos lejos de su alcance.

En caso de envenenamiento, llame al Poison Control Center (Centro Contra Envenenamiento): #_____.

¿Tiene armas en su casa? Si usted necesitara tener un arma (de fuego) en la casa, manténgala descargada, en un lugar seguro y bajo llave. Mantenga las municiones en un lugar diferente a donde guarda el arma.

Nunca deje a su niño sin supervisión cerca del agua, como por ejemplo la bañera, el inodoro o excusado, pozos, piscinas, lagos, u océano.

It is important to use a high-factor sunscreen (SPF 30 or more) on your child when he/she is outdoors.

Es importante aplicarle un aceite bronceador con protector solar de número alto (SPF treinta o mayor) cuando esté en el sol.

Are you concerned about violence in your home or neighborhood?

¿Le preocupa la violencia en su casa o vecindario?

◆ **Immunization & lab considerations**
   (See immunization schedule, Appendix.)

Pb if indicated
PPD if indicated

Hemoglobin or hematocrit if child is at risk

Stage Visit: 2 years

History	**Historia**
◆ **Chief complaint**	◆ **Molestia principal**
What brings you in today?	¿Qué los trae por acá?
Have you brought your child for a routine checkup?	¿Trae a su niño/a para un chequeo de rutina?
How is your child?	¿Cómo está su niño/a?
Do you have any concerns or particular questions?	¿Tiene usted alguna preocupación o pregunta en especial?
Since the last visit, has your child had any illness? Accident? Taken any medicine?	¿Desde la última visita, ha tenido su niño/a alguna enfermedad? ¿Accidente? ¿Recibió alguna medicina?
◆ **Nutrition**	◆ **Nutrición**
Is your child eating well?	¿Come bien su niño/a?
What does he/she eat? How much? What does he/she like most?	¿Qué come él/ella? ¿Cuánto? ¿Qué es lo que más le gusta?
◆ **Behavior**	◆ **Comportamiento**
Does your child seem happy?	¿Le parece alegre su niño/a?
Are you enjoying your child?	¿Disfruta usted a su niño/a?
What do you do together?	¿Qué cosas hacen ustedes juntos?

| Does he/she sleep well? | ¿Duerme bien? |
| Is he/she beginning to toilet train? | ¿Está aprendiendo a usar el baño? |

Development / Desarrollo

What is he/she able to do now?	¿Qué puede hacer él/ella ahora?
Can your child:	¿Puede su niño/a:
walk upstairs?	subir gradas andando?
run?	correr?
throw a ball?	tirar una bola?
put on some clothing?	ponerse la ropa?
turn pages of a book?	voltear las paginas de un libro?
name parts of the body?	nombrar partes del cuerpo?

Physical Exam	Developmental Exam
height, weight	Gross Motor: throw/kick ball, jump
strabismus	Visual Motor: turn single page, put on clothing
vision, hearing	Language: 6 body parts, two-word phrases
teeth	Social: help dressing, may name friend
gait	

Intervention

◆ Instructions

Your child should be eating normal food.

Be careful with foods he/she can choke on.

Do not give:
  peanuts, raisins, whole beans
  large pieces of hot dog

  raw vegetables
  large pieces of fruit

You should brush his/her teeth with just a little toothpaste.

Talk with your child frequently to help him/her learn to speak.

He/she should have a regular bedtime.

He/she should not watch too much television — it is better to play and read with him/her.

Intervención

◆ Instrucciones

Su niño/a debe comer comida normal.

Tenga cuidado con las comidas con las que pueda atragantarse.

No le dé:
  maní, pasas, frijoles enteros
  pedazos grandes de hot dog (salchicha)
  verduras crudas
  pedazos grandes de fruta

Debe cepillar sus dientes con un poquito de pasta dental.

Hable mucho con su niño/a para ayudarle a aprender a hablar.

Su niño/a debe tener una hora fija para acostarse.

No le permita ver mucha televisión — es mejor jugar y leer con él/ella.

◆ Safety

You should use:
- car seats
- smoke detectors in the home
- locks for cabinets and windows
- outlet covers
- stairway gates
- sun protection

Be careful about the hot water temperature. Reduce to 120° to prevent accidental burns.

Caution with pots on the stove. Turn handles so that your child cannot reach them.

Place medications and chemicals out of reach. In case of poisoning, call the Poison Control Center at #_____.

◆ Seguridad

Debe usar:
- una silla para niños en el carro
- detectores de humo en la casa
- seguros para armarios y ventanas
- cubiertas para los toma corriente
- barreras para las escaleras
- protección contra el sol

Tenga cuidado con la temperatura del agua caliente. Rebájela a 120 (ciento veinte) grados para prevenir quemaduras.

Tenga cuidado con ollas encima de la estufa. Voltee los agarraderos para que su niño/a no los alcance.

Ponga medicinas y químicos lejos de su alcance. En caso de envenenamiento, llame al Poison Control Center (Centro Contra Envenenamiento): #_____.

◆ **Safety (continued)**

Do you have any guns in your home? If you need to keep a gun in your house, keep the gun unloaded and locked up. Store the ammunition in a different place away from the gun.

Never leave your child alone near water — a bathtub, toilet, well, swimming pool, lake, or ocean.

It is important to use a high-factor sunscreen (SPF 30 or more) on your child when he/she is outdoors.

◆ **Seguridad (continuación)**

¿Tiene armas en su casa? Si usted necesitara tener un arma (de fuego) en la casa, manténgala descargada, en un lugar seguro y bajo llave. Mantenga las municiones en un lugar diferente a donde guarda el arma.

Nunca deje a su niño sin supervisión cerca del agua, como por ejemplo la bañera, el W.C. (excusado), pozos, piscinas, lagos u océano.

Es importante aplicarle un aceite bronceador con protector solar de número alto (SPF treinta o mayor) cuando esté en el sol.

◆ **Immunization & lab considerations**
     (See immunization schedule, Appendix.)

Cholesterol if indicated
Pb if indicated

PPD if indicated
Hemoglobin or hematocrit if child is at risk

Stage Visit: 3 years

History

◆ **Chief complaint**

What brings you
in today?

Have you brought your
child for a routine
checkup?

How is your child?
To child:

How are you?

Do you have any
concerns or particular
questions?

Since the last visit,
has your child had
any illness?
Accident?
Taken any
medicine?

◆ **Nutrition**

Is your child eating
well?

What does he/she eat?
How much?
What does he/she like
most?

Historia

◆ **Molestia principal**

¿Qué los trae
por acá?

¿Trae a su niño/a
para un chequeo
de rutina?

¿Cómo está su niño/a?

¿Cómo estás?

¿Tiene usted alguna
preocupación o
pregunta en
especial?

¿Desde la última visita,
ha tenido su niño/a
alguna enfermedad?
¿Accidente?
¿Recibió alguna
medicina?

◆ **Nutrición**

¿Come bien su
niño/a?

¿Qué come él/ella?
¿Cuánto?
¿Qué es lo que
más le gusta?

◆ Behavior	**◆ Comportamiento**
Does your child seem happy?	¿Le parece alegre su niño/a?
Does he/she eat/sleep well?	¿Duerme/come bien?
Is he/she toilet trained?	¿Sabe usar el baño?
Is he/she in a preschool program, such as Head Start?	¿Está en un programa preescolar, como Head Start?
To child:	
How do you like school?	¿Te gusta la escuela?
What do you like to do most?	¿Qué te gusta hacer más?
Do you have a best friend?	¿Tienes un/a mejor amigo/a?
Are you learning English?	¿Estás aprendiendo el inglés?

Development	**Desarrollo**
What is he/she able to do now?	¿Qué puede hacer él/ella ahora?
Can your child:	¿Puede su niño/a:
run and play normally?	correr y jugar normalmente?
ride a tricycle?	manejar un triciclo?
dress by him/herself?	vestirse solo/a?
speak fairly clearly?	hablar con bastante claridad?
play/share with other children?	jugar/compartir con otros niños?

To child:

What is your name?

¿Cómo te llamas?

What is your first
name, last name?

¿El nombre,
El apellido?

Can you do (draw)
this? Show me.

¿Puedes hacer
(dibujar) esto?
Muéstrame.

Physical Exam

height, weight

blood pressure

strabismus

hearing, vision

teeth

gait

Developmental Exam

Gross Motor: ride tricycle,
balance 2 seconds,
may hop

Visual Motor: copy circle,
cross

Language: 3-word
sentences, 1+ colors,
speech understandable
to parents

Social: share, rule games,
know name/sex

Intervention

◆ **Instructions**

Your child should be
eating a healthy and
balanced diet.

He/she should begin
learning to brush his/her
own teeth. (He/she will
need your help until
he/she is older.)

Your child should begin
to see a dentist twice
a year.

Intervención

◆ **Instrucciones**

Su niño/a debe comer
una dieta sana y
balanceada.

Debe empezar a
aprender a cepillarse
los dientes. (Va a
necesitar su ayuda
hasta que esté mayor.)

Debe empezar a
visitar al dentista
dos veces al año.

◆ **Instructions (continued)**

He/she should have regular mealtimes and bedtime.

Limit snacking between meals.

He/she should not watch too much television — it is better to play and read with him/her.

Help your child to make choices and develop independence.

Are you enrolling your child in any preschool program?

◆ **Safety**

You should use:

car seats

smoke detectors in the home

locks for cabinets and windows

outlet covers

stairway gates

sun protection

◆ **Instrucciones (continuación)**

Su niño/a debe tener horas fijas para comer y acostarse.

Ne le permita comer demasiado entre comidas.

No le permita ver mucha televisión — es mejor jugar y leer con él/ella.

Ayude a su niño/a a tomar decisiones y desarrollar su independencia.

¿Va a matricular a su niño/a en un programa pre-escolar?

◆ **Seguridad**

Debe usar:

una silla para niños en el carro

detectores de humo en la casa

seguros para armarios y ventanas

cobertores para los toma corrientes

barreras para las escaleras

protección contra el sol

Be careful about the hot water temperature. Reduce to 120° to prevent accidental burns.

Caution with pots on the stove. Turn handles so that your child cannot reach them.

Place medications and chemicals out of reach. In case of poisoning, call the Poison Control Center at #_____.

Do you have any guns in your home? If you need to keep a gun in your house, keep the gun unloaded and locked up. Store the ammunition in a different place away from the gun.

Tenga cuidado con la temperatura del agua caliente. Rebájela a 120 (ciento veinte) grados para prevenir quemaduras.

Tenga cuidado con las ollas encima de la estufa. Voltee los agarradores para que su niño/a no los alcance.

Ponga medicinas y químicos lejos de su alcance. En caso de envenenamiento, llame al Poison Control Center (Centro Contra Envenenamiento): #_____.

¿Tiene armas en su casa? Si usted necesitara tener un arma (de fuego) en la casa, manténgala descargada, en un lugar seguro y bajo llave. Mantenga las municiones en un lugar diferente a donde guarda el arma.

◆ **Safety (continued)**

Never leave your child alone near water — a bathtub, toilet, well, swimming pool, lake, or ocean.

Teach your child not to speak with strangers or to accept food from them.

It is important to use a high-factor sunscreen (SPF 30 or more) on your child when he/she is outdoors.

Teach your child never to cross a street without holding an adult's hand.

Are you concerned about violence in your home or neighborhood?

◆ **Seguridad (continuación)**

Nunca deje a su niño sin supervisión cerca del agua, como por ejemplo la bañera, el W.C. (excusado), pozos, piscinas, lagos, u océano.

Enséñele a su niño a no hablarle a extraños ni a aceptar comida o dulces de extraños.

Es importante aplicarle un aceite bronceador con protector solar de número alto (SPF treinta o mayor) cuando esté en el sol.

Enséñele a su niño a nunca cruzar la calle sin estar agarrado de la mano de un adulto.

¿Le preocupa la violencia en su casa o vecindario?

◆ **Immunization & lab considerations**
   (See immunization schedule, Appendix.)

Cholesterol if indicated
Dental care
Pb if indicated
PPD if indicated

Stage Visit: 4 years

History

◆ Chief complaint

What brings you in today?

Have you brought your child for a routine checkup?

How is your child?

To child:

How are you?

Do you have any concerns or particular questions?

Since the last visit, has your child had any illness? Accident? Taken any medicine?

◆ Nutrition

Is your child eating well?

What does he/she eat? How much? What does he/she like most?

Historia

◆ Molestia principal

¿Qué los trae por acá?

¿Trae a su niño/a para un chequeo de rutina?

¿Cómo está su niño/a?

¿Cómo estás?

¿Tiene usted alguna preocupación o pregunta en especial?

¿Desde la última visita, ha tenido su niño/a alguna enfermedad? ¿Accidente? ¿Recibió alguna medicina?

◆ Nutrición

¿Come bien su niño/a?

¿Qué come él/ella? ¿Cuánto? ¿Qué es lo que más le gusta?

◆ Behavior

Does your child seem happy?

Does he/she sleep well?

Is he/she fully toilet trained?

To child:

Are you in school? Which one? Do you like it?

What do you like to do most?

Do you have a best friend?

Are you learning English?

Development

What is he/she able to do now?

Can your child:
run and play normally?
ride a bicycle/ tricycle?
dress by him/herself?
name colors?
speak in complete sentences?

◆ Comportamiento

¿Le parece alegre su niño/a?

¿Duerme bien?

¿Sabe usar el baño perfectamente?

¿Vas a la escuela? ¿Cuál? ¿Te gusta?

¿Qué te gusta hacer más?

¿Tienes un/a mejor amigo/a?

¿Estás aprendiendo el inglés?

Desarrollo

¿Qué puede hacer él/ella ahora?

¿Puede su niño/a:
correr y jugar normalmente?
manejar bicicleta/ triciclo?
vestirse sin ayuda?
nombrar los colores?
hablar bien en frases completas?

count to 10?

play/share with other children?

To child:

> Can you do (draw) this? Show me.

contar del uno al diez?

jugar/compartir con otros niños?

> ¿Puedes hacer (dibujar) esto? Muéstrame.

Physical Exam

height, weight

blood pressure

strabismus

vision, hearing

teeth

gait

hernias

Developmental Exam

Gross Motor: hop, balance 3 to 5 seconds, heel-toe walk

Visual Motor: button, copy cross, may tie shoes

Language: define words, name 4 colors

Social: play rule games, dress without help

Intervention
◆ **Instructions**

Your child should be eating a healthy and balanced diet.

He/she should brush his/her own teeth. (He/she will need your help until he/she is older.)

Your child should see a dentist twice a year.

He/she should have regular mealtimes and bedtime.

Limit snacking between meals.

He/she should not watch too much television — it's better to play and read with him/her.

Help your child to make choices and develop independence.

When will your child enter school?

Intervención
◆ **Instrucciones**

Su niño/a debe comer una dieta sana y balanceada.

Debe cepillar sus dientes. (Va a necesitar su ayuda hasta que este mayor.)

Debe visitar al dentista dos veces al año.

Su niño/a debe tener horas fijas para comer y acostarse.

No le permita comer demasiado entre comidas.

No le permita ver mucha televisión — es mejor jugar y leer con él/ella.

Ayude a su niño/a a tomar decisiones y desarrollar su independencia.

¿Cuándo entrará su niño/a a la escuela?

◆ Safety

You should use:

    seat belt (+ booster seat)

    smoke detectors in the home

    locks for cabinets and windows

    outlet covers

    stairway gates

    sun protection

Be careful about the hot water temperature. Reduce to 120° to prevent accidental burns.

Caution with pots on the stove. Turn handles so that your child cannot reach them.

Place medications and chemicals out of reach. In case of poisoning, call the Poison Control Center at #_____.

◆ Seguridad

Debe usar:

    el cinturón de seguridad (y booster seat)

    detectores de humo en la casa

    seguros para armarios y ventanas

    cubiertas para los toma corrientes

    barreras para las escaleras

    protección contra el sol

Tenga cuidado con la temperatura del agua caliente. Rebájela a 120 (ciento veinte) grados para prevenir quemaduras.

Tenga cuidado con las ollas encima de la estufa. Voltee los agarraderos para que su niño/a no los alcance.

Ponga medicinas y químicos lejos de su alcance. En caso de envenenamiento, llame al Poison Control Center (Centro Contra Envenenamiento): #_____.

◆ Safety (continued)

Do you have any guns in your home? If you need to keep a gun in your house, keep the gun unloaded and locked up. Store the ammunition in a different place away from the gun.

Teach your child not to speak with strangers or to accept food from them.

Teach your child never to cross a street without holding an adult's hand.

Are you concerned about violence in your home or neighborhood?

◆ Seguridad (continuación)

¿Tiene armas en su casa? Si usted necesitara tener un arma (de fuego) en la casa, manténgala descargada, en un lugar seguro y bajo llave. Mantenga las municiones en un lugar diferente a donde guarda el arma.

Enséñele a su niño a no hablarle a extraños ni a aceptar comida o dulces de extraños.

Enséñele a su niño a nunca cruzar la calle sin estar agarrado de la mano de un adulto.

¿Le preocupa la violencia en su casa o vecindario?

◆ Immunization & lab considerations
(See immunization schedule, Appendix.)

Cholesterol if indicated
Pb if indicated
PPD if indicated

Hemoglobin or hematocrit if child is at risk

Stage Visit: 5 years

History

◆ **Chief complaint**

What brings you in today?

Have you brought your child for a routine checkup?

How is your child?

To child:

How are you?

Do you have any concerns or particular questions?

Since the last visit, has your child had any illness? Accident? Taken any medicine?

◆ **Nutrition**

Is your child eating well?
What does he/she eat?
How much?
What does he/she like most?

Historia

◆ **Molestia principal**

¿Qué los trae por acá?

¿Trae a su niño/a para un chequeo de rutina?

¿Cómo está su niño/a?

¿Cómo estás?

¿Tiene usted alguna preocupación o pregunta en especial?

¿Desde la última visita, ha tenido su niño/a alguna enfermedad? ¿Accidente? ¿Recibió alguna medicina?

◆ **Nutrición**

¿Come bien su niño/a?
¿Qué come él/ella?
¿Cuánto?
¿Qué es lo que más le gusta?

◆ Behavior

Does your child seem happy?

Does he/she sleep well?

Is he/she fully toilet trained?

To child:

Are you in school?
Which one?
Do you like it?

What do you like to do most?

Do you have a best friend?

Are you learning English?

◆ Comportamiento

¿Le parece alegre su niño/a?

¿Duerme bien?

¿Sabe usar el baño perfectamente?

¿Vas a la escuela?
¿Cuál?
¿Te gusta?

¿Qué te gusta hacer más?

¿Tienes un/a mejor amigo/a?

¿Estás aprendiendo el inglés?

Development

What is he/she able
to do now?

Can your child:
    run and play
    normally?
    ride a bicycle?
    dress by him- /herself?
    name colors?
    speak in complete
    sentences?
    count to 10?
    play/share with other
    children?

To child:
    Can you do
    (draw) this?
    Show me.

Desarrollo

¿Qué puede hacer
él/ella ahora?

¿Puede su niño/a:
    correr y jugar
    normalmente?
    manejar bicicleta?
    vestirse sin ayuda?
    nombrar colores?
    hablar bien en
    frases completas?
    contar del uno a diez?
    jugar/compartir
    con otros niños?

    ¿Puedes hacer
    (dibujar) esto?
    Muéstrame.

Physical Exam

height, weight

blood pressure

strabismus

vision, hearing

teeth

gait

Developmental Exam

Gross Motor: hop, balance
3 to 5 seconds, heel-toe
walk

Visual Motor: button,
copy cross, may tie
shoes, print letters

Language: tell story,
name 4 colors, good
articulation

Social: play rule games,
dress without help

Intervention

◆ **Instructions**

Your child should be eating a healthy and balanced diet.

He/she should brush his/her own teeth. (He/she will need your help until he/she is older.)

Your child should see a dentist twice a year.

He/she should have regular mealtimes and bedtime.

Limit snacking between meals.

He/she should not watch too much television — it's better to play and read with him/her.

Help your child to make choices and develop independence.

When will your child enter school?

Intervención

◆ **Instrucciones**

Su niño/a debe comer una dieta sana y balanceada.

Debe cepillar sus dientes. (Va a necesitar su ayuda hasta que esté mayor.)

Debe visitar al dentista dos veces al año.

Su niño/a debe tener horas fijas para comer y acostarse.

No le permita comer demasiado entre comidas.

No le permita ver mucha televisión — es mejor jugar y leer con él/ella.

Ayude a su niño/a a tomar decisiones y desarrollar su independencia.

¿Cuándo entrará su niño/a a la escuela?

◆ Safety

You should use:

    seat belt (+ booster seat)

    smoke detectors in the home

    locks for cabinets and windows

    outlet covers

    stairway gates

    sun protection

Be careful about the hot water temperature. Reduce to 120° to prevent accidental burns.

Caution with pots on the stove. Turn handles so that your child cannot reach them.

Place medications and chemicals out of reach. In case of poisoning, call the Poison Control Center at #_____.

◆ Seguridad

Debe usar:

    el cinturón de seguridad (y booster seat)

    detectores de humo en la casa

    seguros para armarios y ventanas

    cubiertas para los toma corrientes

    barreras para las escaleras

    protección contra el sol

Tenga cuidado con la temperatura del agua caliente. Rebájela a 120 (ciento veinte) grados para prevenir quemaduras.

Tenga cuidado con las ollas encima de la estufa. Voltee los agarraderos para que su niño/a no los alcance.

Ponga medicinas y químicos lejos de su alcance. En caso de envenenamiento, llame al Poison Control Center (Centro Contra Envenenamiento): #_____.

◆ **Safety
(continued)**

Do you have any guns
in your home? If you
need to keep a gun in
your house, keep the
gun unloaded and
locked up. Store the
ammunition in a
different place away
from the gun.

You should always wear
a helmet and protective
padding when roller
blading or skate-
boarding. Also when
riding a bicycle.

Never accept a ride
from a stranger.

Are you concerned
about violence in your
home or neighborhood?

◆ **Seguridad
(continuación)**

¿Tiene armas en su
casa? Si usted
necesitara tener un
arma (de fuego) en la
casa, manténgala
descargada, en un
lugar seguro y bajo
llave. Mantenga las
municiones en un
lugar diferente a
donde guarda el
arma.

Debes usar un casco
y protectores para
rodillas y codos cuando
patines o uses el
skateboard (patinete).
Tambien al usar la
bicicleta.

Nunca aceptes un
paseo con extraños.

¿Le preocupa la
violencia en su casa
o vecindario?

◆ **Immunization & lab considerations**
   (See immunization schedule, Appendix.)

Cholesterol if indicated
PPD if indicated
Pb if indicated
Screening for STDs
if indicated

Stage Visit: 6 to 11 years

History

- **Chief complaint**

  What brings you
  in today?

  Have you brought your
  child for a routine
  checkup?

  How is your child?

  To child:
   How are you?

  Do you have any
  concerns or particular
  questions?

  Since the last visit,
  has your child had
  any illness?
  Accident? Taken
  any medicine?

- **Nutrition**

  Is your child eating
  well?

  What does he/she eat?
  How much?

Historia

- **Molestia principal**

  ¿Qué los trae por
  acá?

  ¿Trae a su niño/a
  para un chequeo
  de rutina?

  ¿Cómo está su niño/a?

   ¿Cómo estás?

  ¿Tiene usted alguna
  preocupación o
  pregunta en especial?

  ¿Desde la última visita,
  ha tenido su niño/a
  alguna enfermedad?
  ¿Accidente? ¿Recibió
  alguna medicina?

- **Nutrición**

  ¿Come bien su
  niño/a?

  ¿Qué come él/ella?
  ¿Cuánto?

◆ **Behavior**

Does your child seem happy?

Are there any problems with his/her behavior?

To child:

Are you learning to speak English?

How are you sleeping?

Development

To child:

Are you in school?

Which one?

Do you like it?

What grade are you in?

Who is your teacher?

Do you like him/her?

What is your favorite subject?

How are your grades?

Do you have a best friend?

Other friends?

What do you do for fun?

After school?

Do you play sports?

◆ **Comportamiento**

¿Le parece alegre su niño/a?

¿Hay algún problema con su comportamiento?

¿Estas aprendiendo el inglés?

¿Duermes bien?

Desarrollo

¿Estás en una escuela?

¿Cuál?

¿Te gusta?

¿En qué grado estás?

¿Quién es tu maestro/a?

¿Te cae bien?

¿Cuál es tu materia favorita?

¿Cómo son tus grados?

¿Tienes un/a mejor amigo/a?

¿Otros amigos?

¿Qué haces para divertirte?

¿Después de la escuela?

¿Haces deportes?

Physical Exam

height, weight

blood pressure

vision, hearing

scoliosis screen, gait

Tanner stage

pelvic exam for girls and STD screening as indicated

Intervention

◆ **Instructions**

Your child should be eating a healthy and balanced diet.

He/she should brush his/her teeth.

Your child should see a dentist twice a year. (When did he/she last see a dentist?)

He/she should have regular mealtimes and bedtime.

Limit snacking between meals.

He/she should not watch too much television.

He/she should get physical exercise regularly.

Intervención

◆ **Instrucciones**

Su niño/a debe comer una dieta sana y balanceada.

Debe cepillar sus dientes.

Debe visitar al dentista dos veces al año. (¿Cuándo fue al dentista por última vez?)

Su niño/a debe tener horas fijas para comer y acostarse.

No le permita comer demasiado entre comidas.

No le permita ver mucha televisión.

Él/ella debe hacer ejercicio regularmente.

◆ Instructions (continued)

He/she should drink adequate amounts of fluids during exercise and sports activities.

Help your child to make choices and develop independence.

◆ Safety

He/she should always use seat belts and a bike helmet. (It's the law.)

Do you have smoke detectors in the home?

In case of poisoning, call the Poison Control Center at #_____.

Do you have any guns in your home? If you need to keep a gun in your house, keep the gun unloaded and locked up. Store the ammunition in a different place away from the gun.

◆ Instrucciones (continuación)

Debe beber cantidades adecuadas de líquidos durante el ejercicio y las actividades deportivas.

Ayude a su niño/a a tomar decisiones y desarrollar su independencia.

◆ Seguridad

Él/ella debe usar siempre el cinturón de seguridad y un casco cuando monte en bicicleta. (Es la ley.)

¿Tienen detectores de humo en la casa?

En caso de envenenamiento, llame al Poison Control Center (Centro Contra Envenenamiento): #_____.

¿Tiene armas en su casa? Si usted necesitara tener un arma (de fuego) en la casa, manténgala descargada, en un lugar seguro y bajo llave. Mantenga las municiones en un lugar diferente a donde guarda el arma.

Teach your child not to speak with strangers or to accept food from them.	Enséñele a su niño a no hablarle a extraños ni a aceptar comida o dulces de extraños.
It is important to use a high-factor sunscreen on your child when he/she is outdoors.	Es importante aplicarle un aceite bronceador con protector solar de número alto cuando esté en el sol.
You should always wear a helmet and protective padding when roller blading or skate-boarding. Also when riding a bicycle.	Debes usar un casco y protectores para rodillas y codos cuando patines o uses el skateboard (patinete). Tambien al usar la bicicleta.
Never accept a ride from a stranger.	Nunca aceptes un paseo con extraños.

◆ Immunization & lab considerations
(See immunization schedule, Appendix.)

Cholesterol if indicated
Hgb/Hct (11 to 21 y)
PPD if indicated
UA (11 to 21 y)
Update immunizations

Stage Visit: 12 to 21 years

History (from parent)	Historia (de los padres)
How is your child?	¿Cómo está su niño/a?
Do you have any concerns or particular questions?	¿Tiene usted alguna preocupación o pregunta?
Since the last visit, has he/she had any illness? Accident? Taken any medication?	¿Desde la última visita, ha tenido alguna enfermedad? ¿Accidente? ¿Ha tomado alguna medicina?
Does your child seem happy?	¿Le parece alegre su niño/a?
Are there any problems with his/her behavior?	¿Hay algún problema con su conducta?
With older children, I always like to speak with them (examine them) for awhile alone.	Con niños mayores, yo suelo hablarles (examinarlos) por un rato a solas.
Could you excuse us for a moment?	¿Podría usted dejarnos por un momento?

History (from adolescent)	Historia (del adolescente)
◆ Chief complaint	◆ Molestia principal
What brings you in today?	¿Qué te trae por acá?
Are you here for a routine checkup?	¿Estás aquí para un chequeo de rutina?
How are you?	¿Cómo estás?

Are there any problems you would like to discuss?

◆ **Nutrition**

What do you eat?

Do you eat three regular meals? Snacks?

Be sure to include foods high in calcium in your diet.

◆ **Behavior**

Are you learning to speak English?

How are you sleeping?

Development & Social (HEADSS)

◆ **Home**

Who lives at home with you?

Do you have any problems with your parents?

How do you get along with your brothers and sisters?

Do you always feel safe at home?

Has anyone ever touched you with sexual intentions?

¿Hay alguna pregunta que quieres hacer?

◆ **Nutrición**

¿Qué comes?

¿Comes tres comidas regulares? ¿Entre comidas?

Cerciórese de incluir en su dieta alimentos ricos en calcio.

◆ **Comportamiento**

¿Estas aprendiendo el inglés?

¿Duermes bien?

Desarrollo y Social (HEADSS)

◆ **Hogar**

¿Quién vive en la casa contigo?

¿Tienes algún problema con tus padres?

¿Te llevas bien con tus hermanos?

¿Te sientes siempre seguro/a en la casa?

¿Alguna vez te ha tocado alguien con intenciones sexuales?

◆ Education

What grade are you in?

How do you like school?

How are your grades?

Do you receive any special help at school?

Is there violence at school? Gangs? Weapons?

◆ Activities

Do you have a best friend?
Other friends?

What do you do for fun?
After school?

Do you play sports?
Which ones?

◆ Drugs

Do your friends drink alcohol?
Smoke cigarettes?
Use drugs?

How about you?

Do you smoke? How many cigarettes per day?

Do you drink alcohol?
Beer, wine, liquor?
How much per week?

◆ Educación

¿En qué grado estás?

¿Te gusta la escuela?

¿Cómo son tus grados?

¿Recibes ayuda especial en la escuela?

¿Hay violencia en la escuela? ¿Pandillas? ¿Armas?

◆ Actividades

¿Tienes un/a mejor amigo/a?
¿Otros amigos?

¿Cómo te diviertes?
¿Después de la escuela?

¿Haces deportes?
¿Cuáles?

◆ Drogas

¿Toman tus amigos alcohol?
¿Fuman cigarrillos?
¿Usan drogas?

¿Y tú?

¿Fumas? ¿Cuántos cigarrillos al día?

¿Tomas alcohol?
¿Cerveza, vino, licor?
¿Cuánto a la semana?

Have you ever used
drugs?
What type? Do you
use them often?

Have you ever used
IV drugs?
Shared needles?

◆ **Sex**

Is there anyone to
whom you are sexually
attracted?

Are you attracted to
men, women, or both?

Have you ever had
questions about your
sexual orientation?

Do you have a
boyfriend/girlfriend?

Have you been
sexually involved
with anyone?

What type of sex?
Intercourse?
Oral? Anal?

Do you want to
become pregnant?

Do you use any type
of contraception?
What? Condoms?
Diaphragm?
Pill?
Depo-Provera?

¿Has probado
drogas alguna vez?
¿Cuál? ¿Las usas
con frecuencia?

¿Te has inyectado
drogas alguna vez?
¿Has compartido
agujas?

◆ **Sexualidad**

¿Hay alguien a quien
te sientes atraído/a
sexualmente?

¿Te gustan los hombres,
las mujeres, o ambos?

¿Has tenido preguntas
alguna vez sobre tu
orientación sexual?

¿Tienes un/a
novio/a?

¿Has estado
involucrado/a
sexualmente con
alguien alguna vez?

¿Qué tipo de sexo
tienes? ¿Coito?
¿Oral? ¿Anal?

¿Quieres quedar
embarazada?

¿Usas algún tipo de
anticonceptivo?
¿Cuál? ¿Condones?
¿Diafragma?
¿La píldora?
¿Depo-Provera?

◆ Sex (continued)

Do you know how to use a condom?

Have you ever had discharge from your penis/vagina?

Have you started menstruating yet? When?

Are you regular? How long between periods?

How many days are your periods?

When did your last period start?

Have you missed any periods?

Do you get cramps? Do they keep you from doing regular activities?

What do you do to relieve them?

Do you have any children? How many?

Have you ever been pregnant?

How many times? When?

◆ Sexualidad (continuación)

¿Sabes cómo usar un condón?

¿Has tenido alguna vez flujo por tu pene/vagina?

¿Ya empezaste a menstruar? ¿Cuándo empezaste?

¿Eres regular? ¿Cuánto tiempo entre períodos (las reglas)?

¿Cuántos días duran los períodos?

¿Cuándo empezó tu último período?

¿Perdiste un período alguna vez?

¿Tienes cólicos fuertes? ¿Interfieren con tus actividades del día?

¿Qué haces para aliviarlos?

¿Tienes hijos? ¿Cuántos?

¿Has estado embarazada alguna vez?

¿Cuántas veces? ¿Cuándo?

Have you ever had a miscarriage?
An abortion?

◆ **Suicide**
What is your mood generally?

Do you ever get very sad? About what?

Have you ever thought about killing yourself? How would you do it?

Have you ever tried to kill yourself?

¿Has tenido alguna vez una pérdida?
¿Un aborto?

◆ **Suicidio**
¿Generalmente cómo está tu estado de ánimo?

¿Te sientes a veces muy triste? ¿Por qué?

¿Has pensado alguna vez en quitarte la vida? ¿Cómo lo harías?

¿Has tratado alguna vez de quitarte la vida?

Physical Exam

height, weight

blood pressure

vision, hearing

scoliosis screen, gait

Tanner stage, pelvic examination if sexually active or 18 years of age or older

Assess girls involved in sports for eating disorders, menstrual dysfunction, and decreased bone mineral density. Assess boys involved in sports for eating disorders.

Intervention
♦ Instructions

Do you know how to resist drugs and alcohol? How do you do it?

Do you use designated drivers when you go to drink with friends?

How much TV do you watch per day?

Do you read at home? How much?

Do you plan to finish high school?

What do you plan to do after high school?

You should learn to examine your breasts/testicles, and you should examine them once every month. If you ever feel any lumps, you should inform your doctor.

Use condoms each time you have sex.

Intervención
♦ Instrucciones

¿Sabes cómo resistir drogas y alcohol? ¿Cómo lo haces tú?

¿Designan a un "chofer" cuando tomas bebidas alcoholicos con tus amigos?

¿Cuánta televisión miras diariamente?

¿Lees en casa? ¿Cuánto?

¿Piensas en acabar la escuela superior?

¿Qué piensas hacer después de la escuela superior?

Debes aprender a examinarte los pechos/testículos, y debes examinarlos una vez al mes. Si sientes alguna masa o bolita debes informarle a tu doctor.

Usa condones cada vez que tengas relaciónes sexuales.

◆ Safety

You should always use a seat belt in a car, and a helmet when you ride a bicycle or motorcycle.

Never drive after you drink, even if you don't feel drunk.

Do not ride in a car if the driver has been drinking.

Do you have any guns in your home?
If you need to keep a gun in your house, keep the gun unloaded and locked up.

Store the ammunition in a different place away from the gun.

You should always wear a helmet and protective padding when roller blading or skateboarding.

Never accept a ride from a stranger.

◆ Seguridad

Siempre debes usar el cinturón de seguridad en el carro y un casco en la bicicleta o en la moto.

Es importante nunca conducir después de beber, aunque no te sientas borracho/a.

No subas a un automóvil si el chofer ha estado bebiendo alcohol.

¿Tienes armas en tu casa?
Si necesitas tener un arma (de fuego) en la casa, manténla descargada, en un lugar seguro y bajo llave.

Mantén las municiones en un lugar diferente a donde guardas el arma.

Debes usar un casco y protectores para rodillas y codos cuando patines o uses el skateboard (patinete).

Nunca aceptes un paseo con extraños.

◆ **Safety
(continued)**

Too much sun will
wrinkle your skin
prematurely.
You should use
high-factor sunscreen
when you are out in
the sun.

◆ **Seguridad
(continuación)**

Demasiado sol va
a arrugar tu piel
prematuramente.
Debes usar aceite
bronceador con
protector solar de
número alto cuando
estés en el sol.

◆ **Immunization & lab considerations**

   (See immunization schedule, Appendix.)

Cholesterol if indicated
Hgb/Hct (11 to 21 y)
Pap, STD screen if
   indicated
PPD if indicated
UA (11 to 21 y)

Target Systems

Constitutional & Hematology/ Oncology

Has he/she/you lost/gained weight? How much? Over how much time?

Is he/she/you growing normally?

Is his/her/your appetite normal, increased, or decreased? Exactly what, and how much, did he/she/you eat today? Yesterday? For breakfast? Lunch? Dinner? Snacks?

Has he/she/you had less energy than usual? Since when? Has he/she/you been sleeping more than usual? How much?

Has he/she/you been playing normally?

Has he/she been unusually irritable? Has he/she seemed sad? Has he/she been crying more than usual?

Constitucional y Hematológico/ Oncológico

¿Ha perdido/ganado peso? ¿Cuánto? ¿En cuánto tiempo?

¿Crece normalmente?

¿Es su apetito normal, aumentado o disminuido? ¿Exactamente qué y cuánto comió hoy? ¿Ayer? ¿En el desayuno? ¿Almuerzo? ¿Cena? ¿Entre comidas?

¿Ha tenido menos energía que la usual? ¿Desde cuándo? ¿Ha estado durmiendo más que lo usual? ¿Cuánto?

¿Juega normalmente?

¿Ha estado inusualmente irritable? ¿Ha parecido triste? ¿Ha llorado más que lo usual?

Constitutional & Hematology/ Oncology
(continued)

Has he/she/you had a fever? Since when? Did you measure it?

By mouth?
By rectum?
How high was it?
Has he/she/you had chills?

Did he/she/you take anything for the fever? What? When?

Has he/she/you had night sweats?

Have you noticed enlarged lymph nodes? Are they tender?

Does he/she/you bruise easily?

Skin

Has he/she/you had any rashes?

Where?
When did the rash start?
Where on the body did the rash start?

Constitucional y Hematológico/ Oncológico
(continuación)

¿Ha tenido fiebre?
¿Desde cuándo?
¿Le tomó la temperatura?
¿Por la boca?
¿Por el recto?
¿Qué tan alta estaba?
¿Ha tenido escalofríos?

¿Tomó algo para la fiebre? ¿Qué? ¿Cuándo?

¿Ha tenido sudores por las noches?

¿Ha notado inflamación de los ganglios? ¿Duelen?

¿Le aparecen moretones fácilmente?

Piel

¿Ha tenido alguna erupción (algún brote)?
¿Dónde?
¿Cuándo comenzó la erupción (el brote)?
¿En qué parte del cuerpo comenzó la erupción?

Did the rash look the same before or has it changed?	¿Se veía la erupción así antes o ha cambiado?
Does it itch? Hurt?	¿Le pica? ¿Le duele?
Is there any other symptom which accompanies the rash?	¿Algún otro síntoma que acompañe la erupción?
fever	fiebre
a cold	un resfrío
pain in the joints	dolor en las articulaciones
Has he/she/you had this rash before?	¿Ha tenido esta erupción alguna vez antes?
Has he/she/you used anything to treat it? What?	¿Usó algo para tratarla? ¿Qué cosa?
Has he/she/you eaten anything different recently?	¿Ha comido algo diferente recientemente?
Has he/she/you been in contact with anyone with chicken pox? A cold?	¿Ha estado en contacto con alguien con varicela? ¿Con un resfrío?
Does anyone else in the family have this rash?	¿Alguien más en la familia tiene esta erupción?
Have you started using any new detergents recently?	¿Ha empezado a usar un nuevo detergente recientemente?
(soap, shampoo, lotion, cream)	(jabón, champú, loción, crema)
Has he/she/you been swimming in any lakes or pools?	¿Ha nadado en algún lago o piscina?

Skin **(continued)**	**Piel** **(continuación)**

Has he/she/you been in the countryside recently?

¿Ha estado en el campo recientemente?

Has he/she/you had any insect bite?
Tick bite?

¿Le ha picado algún insecto?
¿Una garrapata?

Was there any contact with a poisonous plant?

¿Ha habido algún contacto con alguna planta irritante?

HEENT and Neck

Cabeza y Cuello

- ◆ **Head** (See neurological section, pp. 143-147.)

- ◆ **Eyes**

- ◆ **Ojos**

Does he/she/you wear glasses or contact lenses?

¿Usa anteojos o lentes de contacto?

Has he/she/you had any problems seeing?

¿Ha tenido algún problema con la vista?

Does he/she/you have any problems seeing the board at school?

¿Ha tenido problemas viendo el pizarrón en la escuela?

Where does he/she/you sit in the classroom?
Front?
In the middle?
Back?

¿Dónde se sienta en la clase?
¿Al frente?
¿En el medio?
¿Atrás?

Do you have to squint to see?

¿Tiene que guiñar los ojos para ver?

Has he/she/you gotten anything in the eyes?
What? When?

¿Le ha caído algo en los ojos?
¿Qué? ¿Cuándo?

Do his/her/your eyes hurt?	¿Le duelen los ojos?
Itch?	¿Le pican?
Which eye?	¿Qué ojo?
Right? Left?	¿El derecho? ¿El izquierdo? ¿Ambos?
Both?	
When did the problem start?	¿Cuándo comenzó el problema?
Has any pus come from the eye?	¿Le ha salido pus del ojo?
Has he/she/you had contact with anyone with an eye infection?	¿Ha tenido contacto con alguien con una infección del ojo?

◆ **Ears**

◆ **Oídos**

Do his/her/your ears hurt? Which one?	¿Le duelen los oídos? ¿Cuál?
Has he/she/you been tugging at the ears? When did the pain begin?	¿Ha estado tocándose la oreja? ¿Cuándo empezó el dolor?
Has he/she/you had fever? Chills? Discharge from the ear?	¿Ha tenido fiebre? ¿Escalofrios? ¿Secreción del oído?
Has he/she/you had a runny nose? Sore throat? Cough? Fever?	¿Ha tenido mocos? ¿Ardor de garganta? ¿Tos? ¿Fiebre?
Does he/she/you have trouble hearing? Which ear? Since when?	¿Tiene problemas para oír? ¿Que oído? ¿Desde cuándo?
Has he/she/you put anything in the ear?	¿Se ha puesto algún objeto en el oído?

◆ Ears (continued)

Has he/she/you had
ear infections before?
How often?

When was the last
ear infection?
How were they treated?
Antibiotics?
Which one?

Has he/she/you had
any operations on
the ear? Tubes?

Has his/her/your hearing
been tested? When?
What were the
results?

◆ Nose

Does he/she/you have
a runny nose? A cold?

Does he/she/you have
trouble breathing
through the nose?

Does he/she/you
have allergies?
Sinusitis?
Hay fever?

Does he/she/you
have nosebleeds?
How often?
Since when?
How long do they last?

◆ Oídos (continuación)

¿Ha tenido infección
de oído antes?
¿Con qué frecuencia?

¿Cuándo fue la última
infección de oídos?
¿Cómo la han tratado?
¿Antibióticos?
¿Qué antibiótico?

¿Ha tenido alguna
operación en el oído?
¿Tubitos?

¿Le han chequeado
la audición? ¿Cuándo?
¿Cómo fueron los
resultados?

◆ Nariz

¿Tiene mocos?
¿Está resfriado/a?

¿Tiene problemas
para respirar por
la nariz?

¿Tiene alergias?

¿Sinusitis?
¿Fiebre del heno?

¿Le sale sangre
por la nariz?
¿Con qué frecuencia?
¿Desde cuándo?
¿Cuánto tiempo duran?

132

◆ **Mouth and throat**

Does he/she/you have
a sore throat?

To child:

Does it hurt
to swallow?

Can he/she/you
swallow/eat/drink?

Does he/she/you
have a toothache?
Which tooth?

Does he/she/you have
any sores in the mouth?

Has he/she/you been
around anyone with a
sore throat?

Has anyone in the
family had strep
throat?

Has he/she/you had
a runny nose?
Fever? Cough?

Has he/she/you ever
had rheumatic fever?

Has he/she/you had
a tonsillectomy?

◆ **Boca y garganta**

¿Tiene ardor de
garganta?

¿Te duele al
tragar?

¿Puede tragar/
comer/beber?

¿Tiene dolor en
un diente?
¿Cuál?

¿Tiene alguna
llaga en la boca?

¿Ha estado cerca
de alguien con dolor
de garganta?

¿Tiene alguien en la
familia infección
por estreptococo?

¿Ha tenido
mocos?
¿Fiebre? ¿Tos?

¿Ha tenido alguna
vez fiebre reumática?

¿Le han sacado
las amígdalas?

◆ Neck

Does he/she/you have a stiff neck?

Does it hurt when he/she/you moves the neck?

Are there any swollen glands in the neck?

Do they hurt?

Has he/she/you had contact with anyone with tuberculosis?

Has he/she/you been scratched by a cat?

◆ Cuello

¿Tiene rigidez en el cuello?

¿Le duele cuando mueve el cuello?

¿Hay ganglios en el cuello?

¿Le duelen?

¿Ha tenido contacto con alguien con tuberculosis?

¿Le ha arañado algún gato?

Respiratory

Does he/she/you have a:

cough?

runny nose?

sore throat?

earache?

sinusitis?

fever? How high?

Is he/she/you bringing up sputum? What color: white, yellow, green?

Is he/she/you having trouble breathing?
Does it hurt when he/she/you takes a deep breath?

Has he/she/you had contact with anyone with a cold?
Tuberculosis?

Respiratorio

¿Tiene:

tos?

mocos (flujo nasal)?

ardor de garganta?

dolor de oído?

sinusitis?

fiebre? ¿Qué tan alta?

¿Tiene flema?
¿Qué color: blanca, amarilla, verde?

¿Tiene problemas con la respiración?
¿Duele cuando inspiras profundamente?

¿Ha tenido contacto con alguien con un resfrío?

¿Con tuberculosis?

Has he/she/you ever had a positive PPD? (TB test injected into the arm)	¿Ha tenido alguna vez la prueba de PPD positiva? (prueba para la tuberculosis inyectada en el brazo)
Does he/she/you have asthma?	¿Tiene asma?
Has he/she/you been wheezing?	¿Le silba la respiración?
Since when?	¿Desde cuándo?
Is he/she/you normally on any medications?	¿Toma alguna medicina para esto?
Which ones?	¿Cuáles?
How much?	¿Cuánta?
Has he/she/you taken any extra medications today?	¿Ha tomado alguna medicina extra hoy?
Has he/she/you received nebulizers?	¿Lo/a ha nebulizado a su niño/a?
How many?	¿Cuántas veces?
When?	¿Cuándo?
Did he/she/you improve after taking the medication?	¿Mejoró después de tomar la medicina?
What triggered this asthma attack?	¿Qué provocó este ataque de asma?
a cold?	un resfrío?
animals?	animales?
exercise?	ejercicio?
dust?	polvo?
smoke?	humo?
How often does he/she/you get asthma?	¿Con qué frecuencia le da asma?
What triggers it?	¿Qué la provoca?

Respiratory (continued)

Has he/she/you ever been on steroids?

Has he/she/you ever been hospitalized for asthma? Where? When?

Has he/she/you ever been in an ICU? Was he/she/you intubated?

When was his/her/your last emergency room visit for asthma?

How many emergency room visits has he/she/you had this month/year?

Does anyone smoke at home?

Are there pets?

Is it very dusty? Does anyone else in the family have asthma? Eczema? Hay fever?

Respiratorio (continuación)

¿Ha recibido alguna vez esteroides?

¿Ha estado hospitalizado/a alguna vez? ¿Dónde? ¿Cuándo?

¿Ha estado alguna vez en la unidad de cuidados intensivos? ¿Fue intubado/a?

¿Cuándo fue su última visita a la sala de emergencia por asma?

¿Cuántas veces ha estado en la sala de emergencia este mes/año?

¿Fuma alguien en la casa?

¿Hay animales?

¿Hay mucho polvo? ¿Hay alguien más en la familia con asma? ¿Eczema? ¿Fiebre del heno?

Cardiovascular

Have you ever been told that he/she/you has a heart problem?

Has he/she/you ever had a heart murmur?

Has he/she/you ever had any special tests for the heart?
EKG? Echocardiogram (ultrasound of the heart)?

Has he/she/you ever had palpitations (unusually fast and strong heartbeats)?
Chest pain?
Has he/she/you ever passed out?
What happened?
Has he/she/you ever felt dizzy with exercise?
Did he/she/you pass out?

Can he/she/you keep up with friends when playing sports?
Did anyone in the family die young of heart problems?
How old was he/she?
What did he/she have?

Cardiovascular

¿Alguna vez le han dicho que tiene problemas con el corazón?

¿Ha tenido alguna vez un soplo cardíaco?

¿Le han hecho alguna vez un exámen especial para el corazón?
¿Electrocardiograma?
¿Ecocardiograma (ultrasonido del corazón)?

¿Has tenido alguna vez palpitaciones (latidos muy rápidos y fuertes)?
¿Dolor en el pecho?
¿Te has desmayado alguna vez?
¿Qué pasó?
¿Se ha sentido alguna vez mareado/a haciendo ejercicio?
¿Se desmayó?

¿Puede él/ella jugar deportes como sus amigos?
¿Murió alguien en la familia muy joven del corazón?
¿De que edad?
¿Qué tuvo?

Gastrointestinal

Has he/she/you been vomiting? How many times? Since when?
Does he/she/you vomit with tremendous force? How far?

What does the vomit look like? Is there any blood? Is it yellow? Green?

Does he/she/you have any stomach pain? Where?
How often?
When did it start?
How is the pain?
Sharp? Burning, crampy, gassy?

Does the pain go anywhere — upward, toward the back? What brings on the pain?

Does food make the pain better or worse?

Has he/she/you been eating/drinking?
Does anything relieve the pain? Milk, antacids, stooling?
Does he/she/you get the pain when anxious?

Has he/she/you ever been treated for the pain? How?

Gastrointestinal

¿Ha estado vomitando?
¿Cuántas veces?
¿Desde cuándo?
¿Vomita con gran fuerza?
¿A qué distancia?

¿Cómo es el vómito?
¿Hay sangre?
¿Está amarillo?
¿Verde?

¿Tiene dolores de estómago?
¿Dónde?
¿Con qué frecuencia?
¿Cuándo empezó?
¿Cómo es el dolor?
¿Agudo? ¿Como ardor, calambres, gas?

¿Se va el dolor hacia alguna parte — arriba, a la espalda?
¿Qué ocasiona el dolor?

¿Con la comida, mejora o empeora el dolor?

¿Ha estado comiendo, bebiendo?
¿Hay algo que alivie el dolor? ¿La leche, antiácidos, evacuación?
¿Le dá el dolor cuando está nervioso/a?

¿Alguna vez le han tratado el dolor?
¿Cómo?

English	Spanish
When was his/her/your last bowel movement? What did the stool look like?	¿Cuándo evacuó por ultima vez? ¿Cómo eran las heces?
Has he/she/you had diarrhea? Since when? How many times per day? Are the stools watery or just soft? What color? Is there mucus, blood, worms?	¿Ha tenido diarrea? ¿Desde cuándo? ¿Cuántas veces al día? ¿Son las heces aguadas o solamente suaves? ¿De que color? ¿Hay moco, sangre, lombrices?
Has he/she/you had any fevers? How high?	¿Ha tenido fiebre? ¿Qué tan alta?
Has he/she/you had any belly pain? Where?	¿Ha tenido dolor de estómago? ¿Dónde?
Has he/she/you eaten anything unusual?	¿Ha comido algo inusual?
Has he/she/you been in contact with sick people?	¿Ha tenido contacto con gente enferma?
Has he/she/you traveled recently?	¿Ha viajado recientemente?
Is he/she/you drinking fluids? How much?	¿Esta tomando líquido? ¿Cuanto?
How many times per day does he/she/you urinate? (wet diapers)	¿Cuántas veces al día orina? (pañales mojados)
Is he/she/you eating? What?	¿Está comiendo bien? ¿Qué come?

Genitourinary	Genitourinario
How many times per day does he/she/you urinate?	¿Cuántas veces al día orina?
How many wet diapers per day?	¿Cuántos pañales moja al día?
Does he/she/you urinate a lot or a little?	¿Orina gran cantidad o poca?
What does the urine look like? Clear, yellow, cloudy, red?	¿Cómo es la orina? ¿Clara, amarilla, turbia, roja?
Does it hurt when he/she/you urinates?	¿Le duele cuando orina?
Does he/she/you cry?	¿Llora?
Is he/she/you urinating more frequently than normal?	¿Está orinando con más frecuencia que lo usual?
Does he/she/you have to get up at night to urinate?	¿Tiene que despertarse en la noche para orinar?
Is this new?	¿Es nuevo esto?
Since when?	¿Desde cuándo?
Does he/she/you leak urine (more than normal)?	¿Se le sale la orina (más que lo usual)?
Has he/she/you ever had a UTI before?	¿Alguna vez ha tenido una infección urinaria?
Do you tend to get them after intercourse?	¿Le dan infecciones después de tener relaciones sexuales?
Does he/she/you have any urinary tract abnormality?	¿Tiene alguna anormalidad del tracto urinario?
Does anyone in the family have kidney disease?	¿Tiene alguien en la familia algún problema con los riñones?

Does he/she/you have any penile/vaginal discharge?	¿Tiene secreción del pene/flujo de la vagina?
What color is it? white, yellow, green, brown, red?	¿Qué color es el flujo? blanco, amarillo, verde, café, rojo?
Does the discharge smell bad, fishy?	¿Huele mal, a pescado?
Does it itch/hurt down below?	¿Le pica/duele abajo?
Are there any open sores?	¿Tiene alguna llaga?
Have you ever had a yeast infection?	¿Ha tenido alguna vez una infección vaginal por cándida?
Have you been sexually active?	¿Es sexualmente activo/a?
When was the last time you had intercourse?	¿Cuándo tuviste sexo por ultima vez?
How many partners have you had?	¿Cuántas parejas has tenido?
Do you use condoms?	¿Usas condones?
Have you ever had an STD? Herpes, gonorrhea, chlamydia, syphilis, pelvic inflammatory disease?	¿Has tenido alguna enfermedad venérea alguna vez? ¿Herpes, gonorrea, clamidia, sífilis, enfermedad inflamatoria pélvica?
Have you had fever? Abdominal pain?	¿Has tenido fiebre? ¿Dolor de abdomen?
Is there any chance you could be pregnant?	¿Hay alguna posibilidad que estés embarazada?

141

Genitourinary (continued)

When was your last period?

Is there any chance that he/she was sexually abused? By whom?

Do you always feel (sexually) safe at home?

Genitourinario (continuación)

¿Cuándo fue su último período?

¿Hay alguna posibilidad que él/ella haya sido maltratado/a sexualmente? ¿Por quién?

¿Te sientes siempre seguro/a (sexualmente) en casa?

(See abuse screening section, pp. 180-181)

Musculoskeletal

How did this happen? Show me.
Did he/she/you hurt anything else?
Has he/she/you ever hurt this before?

We will get an X-ray. It looks like a sprain, broken bone.

Do his/her/your joints hurt? Which ones?

Did he/she/you bump or hurt this joint?
Does he/she/you walk with a limp?
Have the joints ever been (hot, red, swollen, painful) before?

Musculoesquelético

¿Cómo pasó esto? Muéstreme.
¿Se lastimó algo más?
¿Se ha lastimado esta parte alguna vez antes?

Vamos a tomar radiografías. Parece una esguince, fractura.

¿Le duelen las articulaciones? ¿Cuáles?

¿Se golpeó o lastimó esta articulación? ¿Cojea?

¿Han estado las articulaciones (calientes, rojas, hinchadas, dolorosas) alguna vez antes?

Has he/she/you had any rash, fever, insect bites?

¿Ha tenido alguna erupción, fiebre, picadura de un insecto?

Has he/she/you had a sore throat? Discharge from penis, vagina?

¿Ha tenido ardor de garganta? ¿Secreción por el pene, la vagina?

Neurological

◆ **General**

Has he/she/you had any trauma to the head? Falls? Accidents?

Did he/she/you lose consciousness? For how long? When? Has he/she/you ever lost consciousness before? When?

Are you feeling dizzy? Do you feel like the room is spinning?

Do you feel like fainting?

Has he/she/you ever fainted?

Does the dizziness increase when he/she/you stands up?

Neurológico

◆ **General**

¿Ha tenido algún golpe en la cabeza? ¿Caídas? ¿Accidentes?

¿Perdió la consciencia? ¿Por cuánto tiempo? ¿Cuándo? ¿Alguna vez antes tuvo pérdida de consciencia? ¿Cuándo?

¿Se siente mareado/a? ¿Siente como si el cuarto da vueltas?

¿Siente como si estuviera a punto de desmayarse?

¿Se ha desmayado alguna vez?

¿Aumenta el mareo al pararse?

Seizures	Convulsiones
◆ **Seizures**	◆ **Convulsiones**
Did he/she/you have a seizure?	¿Ha tenido algún ataque/convulsión?
What was it like?	¿Cómo fue?
Did he/she/you have a fever at the time?	¿Tuvo fiebre en ese momento?
How high?	¿Qué tan alta?
Did the seizure begin in one place on his/her/your body?	¿Comenzó el ataque en algún lugar del cuerpo?
How long did the seizure last?	¿Cuánto duró?
Was he/she/you confused/unconscious afterwards?	¿Estuvo confuso/a después?
For how long?	¿Por cuánto tiempo?
Was he/she/you incontinent of urine? Stool?	¿Se orinó o defecó?
Has he/she/you had seizures in the past?	¿Ha tenido ataques en el pasado?
Since when?	¿Desde cuándo?
How often?	¿Con qué frecuencia?
Do the seizures occur only with fever?	¿Le dan las convulsiones solamente cuando tiene fiebre?
Does he/she/you have a diagnosed cause of seizures?	¿Le han diagnosticado alguna causa a los ataques?
Does he/she/you take any medications for seizures? In the past?	¿Toma alguna medicina para los ataques? ¿En el pasado?
Which ones?	¿Cuales?

◆ **Headaches**

Do you have a
headache now?
Where is the pain?

Do you get headaches
regularly?
How often?
At what time of day?
Is the pain always in
the same place?

Since when has
he/she/you been
getting headaches?
What usually brings
on the headache?
How long do they
usually last?

Does he/she/you cry
with the headaches?
Do the headaches wake
him/her/you up at night?

Is the pain throbbing
or constant?
Does he/she/you feel
nauseated or has
he/she/you vomited?
Does he/she/you see
lights or notice any
change in vision before
the headache begins?

◆ **Dolores de cabeza**

¿Tienes dolor de cabeza
en este momento?
¿Dónde está el dolor?

¿Te dan dolores de
cabeza con regularidad?
¿Con qué frecuencia?
¿En que momento del día?
¿Son siempre en
el mismo lugar?

¿Desde cuándo
tiene los
dolores?
¿Qué provoca el
dolor usualmente?
¿Cuánto tiempo
duran?

¿Llora con el dolor?

¿Le despiertan por
la noche?

¿El dolor es pulsatil
o constante?
¿Siente nausea
o ha vomitado
alguna vez?
¿Vé luces o tiene
algún cambio en la
visión antes que
empieze el dolor?

◆ **Headaches (continued)**

What makes the pain better/worse?
Does he/she/you take medication? What? Does it help?
Do bright lights or loud noises make it worse?

◆ **Sensory**

Is he/she/you having trouble seeing? Hearing?

Where do you sit in class? In the front? Back? Middle?

Do you have trouble seeing what the teacher writes on the blackboard?
Do you have to squint to see?
Do you wear glasses? A hearing aid?
Has he/she/you felt numbness or tingling in hands or feet?

◆ **Dolores de cabeza (continuación)**

¿Que mejora/empeora el dolor?
¿Toma medicina? ¿Qué?
¿Le ayuda?
¿Lo empeoran las luces brillantes o ruidos fuertes?

◆ **Sensorial**

¿Tiene problemas con la vista?
¿El oído?

¿Dónde se sienta en la clase? ¿Al frente? ¿Atrás? ¿En el medio?

¿Tiene problemas para ver lo que escribe la maestra en el pizarrón?
¿Tiene que guiñar los ojos para ver?
¿Usa anteojos?
¿Un audífono?
¿Ha sentido adormecimiento u hormigueos en las manos o pies?

146

◆ **Motor/Coordination**

Can he/she/you crawl/ walk/run/play normally?

Does he have a limp?

Has he/she/you had any loss of balance?

◆ **Speech/Behavior**

Has he/she been acting normally?
Has he/she/you had any trouble speaking?

◆ **Motor/Coordinación**

¿Puede gatear/ caminar/correr/jugar normalmente?

¿Cojea al caminar?

¿Ha tenido pérdida del equilibrio?

◆ **Lenguaje/ Comportamiento**

¿Ha estado actuando con normalidad?
¿Ha tenido algún problema al hablar?

Emergency Department Visit

Brief ED History

Historia Abreviada de Emergencia

◆ Introduction
Hello. My name
is _____.

I am a doctor,
medical student,
nurse.

What is his/her name?
(What is your name?)
How old is he/she/you?

◆ Introducción
Hola. Mi nombre
es _____.

Soy un/a doctor/a,
estudiante de medicina,
enfermero/a.

¿Cómo se llama él/ella?
(¿Cómo te llamas?)
¿Qué edad tiene?
(or: ¿Cuántos años
tiene?)

◆ Chief complaint
What brings you to
the ED?
(What happened?)
Was he/she/you healthy
until now?
Has this ever happened
before?
Is anyone else sick
at home?

◆ Molestia principal
¿Qué les trae
por acá?
(¿Qué pasó?)
¿Ha estado sano/a
hasta ahora?
¿Ha pasado esto
antes?
¿Está alguien enfermo
en la casa?

◆ Past medical history

Birth

When was your child born?

Was he/she born near the due date?

Early, late?

How much did he/she weigh at birth?

Were there any problems with the pregnancy or delivery?

Was he/she born vaginally or by cesarean? Why?

After how many days did he/she leave the hospital?

Medical history

Has he/she/you ever had any serious medical problems?

Has he/she/you ever been hospitalized? For what?

Surgical history

Has he/she/you ever had surgery?

Has he/she/you ever been seriously injured?

◆ Historia médica

Nacimiento

¿Cuándo nació su niño/a?

¿Nació en el tiempo esperado?

¿Fue prematuro/a, tarde?

¿Cuánto pesó al nacer?

¿Hubo problemas durante el embarazo o el parto?

¿Fue un parto vaginal o por cesárea? ¿Por qué?

¿A los cuántos días de nacido dejó el hospital?

Historia médica

¿Ha tenido algún problema médico serio?

¿Ha estado alguna vez hospitalizado/a? ¿Por qué?

Historia quirúrgica

¿Ha tenido alguna operación?

¿Ha tenido alguna herida seria?

Medications
Is he/she/you on any medications? Which?
What dose?
When was the last dose?

Allergies
Is he/she/you allergic to any medications?

Habits
Do you smoke?
Drink alcohol?
Use drugs?
Which?

Travel
Has he/she/you traveled abroad recently?
Where?
When?

Family History
Do any diseases run in the family?

Social History
Where are you from?
Who lives at home with you?

Medicación
¿Toma alguna medicina? ¿Cuáles?
¿En qué dosis?
¿Cuándo fue la última dosis?

Alergias
¿Es alérgico/a a alguna medicina?

Habitos
¿Fumas?
¿Tomas alcohol?
¿Usas alguna droga?
¿Cuáles?

Viajes
¿Ha viajado fuera del país recientemente?
¿Adónde?
¿Cuándo?

Historia familiar
¿Hay alguna enfermedad en la familia?

Historia social
¿De dónde son ustedes?¿Quien vive en casa con ustedes?

Brief ED Scenarios

(See Target System sections for more detail.)

1. **Fever/URI/Earache**
2. **Rashes**
3. **Eye Complaints**
4. **Respiratory Distress**
5. **Asthma**
6. **Vomiting & Diarrhea**
7. **Abdominal Pain**
8. **Headache**
9. **Seizure**
10. **Poisoning**
11. **Trauma: Falls**
12. **Trauma: Motor Vehicle Accident (MVA)**
13. **Trauma: Musculoskeletal**

Situaciones de la Emergencia

1. **Fever/URI/Earache**

   Has he/she/you had a fever?
   Since when?
   Did you measure it?
   By mouth, rectum, under arm?
   How high was it?

   Has he/she/you had:
      chills?
      rash?

      any pain?
      ear pain?
      headache?
      sore throat?

1. **Fiebre/Resfrio/ Dolor de Oídos**

   ¿Ha tenido fiebre?
   ¿Desde cuándo?
   ¿Le tomó la temperatura?
   ¿Por la boca, el recto, debajo del brazo?
   ¿Cuán alta estaba?

   ¿Ha tenido:
      escalofríos?
      una erupción?
      un sarpullido?
      dolor en alguna parte?
      dolor de oído?
      dolor de cabeza?
      dolor de garganta?

1. Fever/URI/Earache (continued)

Has he/she/you had:
 runny nose?
 What color (clear, yellow, green)?

 cough, dry or with phlegm?
 difficulty breathing?

 noisy breathing?
 difficulty swallowing?
 nausea, vomiting?
 diarrhea?
 abdominal pain?
 pain on urination?
 a limp?

Does he/she touch or pull on his/her ear? Which one?

Has he/she seemed tired, irritable?

How is he/she eating, drinking?

Did he/she/you take any medicine? What? When?

Is anyone else in the family sick?

1. Fiebre/Resfrio/ Dolor de Oídos (continuación)

¿Ha tenído:
 mocos?
 ¿De que color (como agua, amarillo, verde)?

 tos, seca o con flema?
 dificultad para respirar?

 respiración ruidosa?
 dificultad para tragar?
 nausea, vómitos?
 diarrea?
 dolor de estómago?
 dolor al orinar?
 cojera?

¿Se toca o jala la oreja? ¿Cuál?

¿Ha estado cansado/a, irritable?

¿Cómo está comiendo, bebiendo?

¿Tomó alguna medicina? ¿Qué? ¿Cuándo?

¿Alguien más está enfermo en la familia?

2. Rashes

Does he/she/you have a rash?
When did it start?
Where did it start exactly?
Has it changed? How?
Has he/she/you been itching?

Has he/she/you had a fever, cough, runny nose?

Has he/she/you had this rash before?

Has he/she/you taken any medications, new foods? Is he/she/you using new soaps, shampoos, deodorant, laundry detergents?

Has he/she/you received immunizations in the last few weeks?

Has he/she/you had chicken pox before?
Has he/she/you been near anyone with chicken pox or a similar rash?

2. Erupciones

¿Tiene alguna erupción?
¿Cuando comenzó?
¿Donde comenzó exactamente?
¿Ha cambiado la erupción? ¿Como?
¿Le dá picazón?

¿Ha tenido fiebre, tos, o mocos?

¿Ha tenido esta erupción antes?

¿Tomó algún medicamento o comida nueva? ¿Esta usando un nuevo champú, desodorante, jabón o detergente?

¿Ha recibido alguna vacuna en las últimas semanas?

¿Ha tenido varicela antes?
¿Ha tenido contacto con alguien con varicela o una erupción similar?

2. Rashes (continued)	**2. Erupciones (continuación)**
Has he/she/you had any insect bites, or been in the country-side?	¿Le ha picado algún insecto, o ha estado en el campo?
Has he/she/you used anything to treat it? What?	¿Ha usado algo para curarla? ¿Que?
3. Eye Complaints	**3. Molestias en los Ojos**
Has he/she/you been rubbing the eyes?	¿Se ha estado frotando los ojos?
Do your eyes hurt?	¿Te duelen los ojos?
Itch?	¿Te pican?
Which eye?	¿Qué ojo?
Right?	¿El derecho?
Left?	¿El izquierdo?
Both?	¿Ambos?
When did the problem start?	¿Cuándo comenzó el problema?
Has he/she/you gotten anything in the eyes? What? When?	¿Le ha entrado algo en los ojos? ¿Qué? ¿Cuándo?
Has he/she/you been hit in the eye?	¿Ha sido golpeado en el ojo?
Does he/she/you have any problems seeing the board at school?	¿Ha tenido problemas viendo el pizarrón en la escuela?
Has any pus come from the eye? What color?	¿Le ha salido pus del ojo? ¿De que color?
Has he/she/you had contact with anyone with an eye infection?	¿Ha tenido contacto con alguien con una infección del ojo?

154

4. Respiratory Distress

Is he/she/you having
trouble breathing?
Since when?

Did it come on
gradually or suddenly?

Can he/she/you eat,
drink, talk, play?
Has he/she/you had
this problem before?
When?

What happened?
Does he/she/you have
a history of asthma?
(see next section)

Has he/she/you had
a fever, cough,
runny nose?

What does the cough
sound like?
Is it barking?

Did he/she put
anything in his/her
mouth? What? When?

Did the problem start
immediately
afterwards?
Is the problem
worse at night?

Has he/she/you had
contact recently
with sick people?

4. Dificultad Respiratoria

¿Tiene alguna
dificultad para respirar?
¿Desde cuándo?

¿Empezó gradualmente
o rápidamente?

¿Puede comer, tomar,
hablar, jugar?
¿Ha tenido este
problema antes?
¿Cuando?

¿Qué pasó?
¿Ha tenido asma?

¿Ha tenido fiebre,
tos, o mocos?

¿Que sonido tiene
la tos?
¿Es cómo una tos
perruna?

¿Se puso algo
en la boca?
¿Qué? ¿Cuándo?

¿Empezó el problema
inmediatamente
después?
¿Empeora el problema
por la noche?

¿Ha tenido
contacto con
alguien enfermo?

4. Respiratory Distress (continued)	4. Dificultad Respiratoria (continuación)

4. **Respiratory Distress (continued)**

Is he/she/you taking any medication?

Does anyone else in the family have this type of problem?

4. **Dificultad Respiratoria (continuación)**

¿Está tomando medicamentos?

¿Hay alguien en la familia con el mismo problema?

5. **Asthma**

When did this attack start?
What brought on this attack?
A cold, exercise, contact with animals/dust?

What medications does he/she/you take normally?

What medications has he/she/you had since this attack started?

How many nebulizers has he/she/you had recently?
Where? When?

What generally brings on the asthma?

Has he/she/you ever been hospitalized for asthma?
Where? When?

5. **Asma**

¿Cuándo empezó este ataque?
¿Qué provocó este ataque?
¿Un resfrío, ejercicio, contacto con animales/polvo?

¿Qué medicinas toma normalmente?

¿Qué medicinas ha tomado desde que comenzó este ataque?

¿Cuántas veces ha usado el nebulizador (la máquina) recientemente?
¿Dónde? ¿Cuándo?

¿Qué provoca su asma normalmente?

¿Ha estado hospitalizado/a alguna vez?
¿Dónde? ¿Cuándo?

Has he/she/you ever been on steroids for asthma?	¿Ha recibido él/ella/usted alguna vez esteroides para el asma?
Has he/she/you ever been in an ICU? Was he/she/you intubated?	¿Ha estado alguna vez en la unidad de cuidados intensivos? ¿Fue intubado/a?
When was your last emergency department visit for asthma?	¿Cuándo era su última visita de servicio de urgencias pasada para el asma?
How many emergency department visits have you had this month/year?	¿Cuántas las visitas de servicio urgencias usted han tenido este mes/año?

6. Vomiting & Diarrhea 6. Vómitos y Diarrea

Has he/she/you been vomiting? How many times? Since when?	¿Ha estado vomitando? ¿Cuántas veces? ¿Desde cuándo?
Does he/she/you vomit with tremendous force?	¿Vomita con gran fuerza?
How far? What does the vomit look like? Is there any blood? Is it green? Is it yellow?	¿A qué distancia? ¿Cómo es el vómito? ¿Hay sangre? ¿Es verde? ¿Es amarillo?

6. Vomiting & Diarrhea (continued)

Does he/she/you have diarrhea?

When did the diarrhea start?

How many stools per day?

How many today? Yesterday?

How many stools normally?

Are the stools watery, thick liquid, or soft?

Is there any mucus, blood? worms?

Has he/she/you had any fevers?

How high?

Has he/she/you been vomiting?

How often?

Has he/she/you had any belly pain?

Where?

Has he/she/you eaten anything new?

Has he/she/you been in contact with sick people?

6. Vómitos y Diarrea (continuación)

¿Tiene diarrea?

¿Cuándo empezó la diarrea?

¿Cuántas veces evacua al día?

¿Cuántas veces hoy? ¿Ayer?

¿Cuántas veces evacua normalmente?

¿Son las heces aguadas, espesas, o suaves?

¿Hay moco, sangre? lombrices?

¿Ha tenido fiebre?

¿Cuán alta?

¿Ha estado vomitando?

¿Con qué frecuencia?

¿Ha tenido dolor de estómago?

¿Dónde?

¿Ha comido algo nuevo?

¿Ha tenido contacto con alguien enfermo?

Has he/she/you traveled recently? Where?	¿Ha viajado recientemente? ¿Adónde?
Is he/she/you drinking fluids? How much today? Yesterday?	¿Está bebiendo líquido? ¿Cuánto hoy? ¿Ayer?
Is he/she/you eating? What?	¿Está comiendo? ¿Qué?
Is he/she/you making urine? How often?	¿Está orinando bien? ¿Con qué frecuencia?
How many wet diapers today? Yesterday? Normally?	¿Cuántos pañales mojó hoy? ¿Ayer? ¿Normalmente?
Is he/she playful, tired, irritable?	¿Le parece su niño/a juguetón/a, cansado/a, irritable?
Has he/she/you taken any medication?	¿Ha tomado alguna medicina?

7. Abdominal Pain   7. Dolor Abdominal

When did the pain start?	¿Cuándo empezó el dolor?
Did it start suddenly or gradually? Where?	¿Empezó de repente o gradualmente? ¿Dónde?
Where is the pain now?	¿Dónde está el dolor ahora?
What is the pain like?	¿Cómo es el dolor?

7. Abdominal Pain (continued)

Is the pain:

 constant?

 dull?

 sharp?

 burning?

 like pressure?

 crampy?

 gassy?

Does it come and go?

Is there anything which brings on the pain (makes it better)?

What makes the pain worse?

Is the pain changing?

Is the pain getting worse (better)?

Has he/she/you had a fever, vomiting, diarrhea?

How many times has he/she/you had vomiting (diarrhea)? When?

How is his/her/your appetite?

When was his/her/your last bowel movement?

7. Dolor Abdominal (continuación)

¿Es el dolor:

 constante?

 sordo?

 agudo?

 ardiente?

 como presión?

 como un calambre?

 como gas?

¿Va y viene?

¿Hay algo que ocasiona (alivia) el dolor?

¿Qué empeora el dolor?

¿Está cambiando el dolor?

¿Está empeorando (mejorando) el dolor?

¿Ha tenido fiebre, vómitos, diarrea?

¿Cuantas veces ha vomitado (evacuado)? ¿Cuando?

¿Cómo está su apetito?

¿Cuándo fue su última evacuación?

Has he/she/you had this pain before? When?	¿Ha tenido este dolor alguna vez antes? ¿Cuándo?
Has he/she/you eaten anything different recently?	¿Ha comido algo diferente recientemente?
Has he/she/you been in contact with anyone who was sick?	¿Ha tenido contacto con alguien enfermo?
Has he/she/you had any abdominal or chest trauma?	¿Ha tenido algún trauma o golpe en el abdomen o el pecho?

8. Headache

8. Cefalea

Do you have a headache now?	¿Tienes dolor de cabeza en este momento?
Where is the pain?	¿Dónde está el dolor?
Do you get headaches regularly? How often?	¿Te dan dolores de cabeza con regularidad? ¿Con qué frecuencia?
At what time of day?	¿En que momento del día?
Is the pain always in the same place?	¿El dolor es siempre en el mismo lugar?
Since when has he/she/you been getting headaches?	¿Desde cuándo tiene los dolores?
What usually brings on the headache?	¿Qué provoca el dolor normalmente?
How long do they usually last?	¿Cuánto tiempo duran?
Does he/she/you cry with the headaches?	¿Llora con el dolor?

161

8. Headache (continued)

Do the headaches wake him/her/you up at night?

Has he/she/you fallen or been hit in the head?

Is the pain throbbing or constant?

Does he/she/you feel nauseated or has he/she/you vomited?

Does he/she/you see lights or notice any change in vision before the headache begins?

Does he/she/you have any changes in gait or weakness?

What makes the pain better/worse?

Does he/she/you take medication? What? Does it help?

Do bright lights or loud noises make it worse?

8. Cefalea (continuación)

¿Lo despiertan por la noche?

¿Se ha caído o ha sufrido un golpe en la cabeza?

¿El dolor es constante o pulsátil?

¿Siente nausea o ha vomitado alguna vez?

¿Vé luces o tiene algún cambio en la visión antes que empiece el dolor?

¿Ha tenido algún cambio en la marcha o debilidad?

¿Qué mejora/empeora el dolor?

¿Toma alguna medicina? ¿Qué? ¿Le ayuda?

¿Lo empeoran las luces brillantes o ruidos fuertes?

9. Seizure

Did he/she/you have a seizure?
What was it like?

Did he/she/you have a fever at the time?
How high?

Did the seizure begin in one place on his/her/your body?

How long did the seizure last?

Was he/she/you confused afterwards?
For how long?

Was he/she/you incontinent of urine?
Stool?

Has he/she/you had seizures in the past?
Since when?
How often?

Do the seizures occur only with fever?

Does he/she/you have a diagnosed seizure disorder?
Epilepsy?

9. Convulsiones

¿Ha tenido algún ataque/convulsión?
¿Cómo fue?

¿Tuvo fiebre en ese momento?
¿Qué tan alta?

¿Comenzó el ataque en algún lugar del cuerpo?

¿Cuánto duró?

¿Estuvo confuso/a después?
¿Por cuánto tiempo?

¿Se orinó o defecó?

¿Ha tenido ataques en el pasado?
¿Desde cuándo?
¿Con qué frecuencia?

¿Le ocurren las convulsiones solamente cuando tiene fiebre?

¿Le han encontrado alguna causa a los ataques?
¿Epilepsia?

9. Seizure (continued)

Does he/she/you take any medications for seizures? In the past?

Has he/she/you ever had trauma to the head?

Has he/she/you ever lost consciousness?

Does anyone in the family have seizures?

10. Poisoning

What did he/she/you swallow? When?

How much did he/she/you swallow?

Do you have the bottle/box?

Has he/she/you vomited?
Did you give him/her/you any treatment?
Charcoal?
Ipecac?
How has he/she/you been acting since this occurred?

9. Convulsiones (continuación)

¿Toma alguna medicina para los ataques? ¿Ha tomado en el pasado?

¿Ha tenido trauma en la cabeza?

¿Perdió la consciencia alguna vez?

¿Hay alguien en la familia que tenga ataques/convulsiones?

10. Envenenamientos

¿Qué se tragó? ¿Cuándo?

¿Cuánto tragó de esto?

¿Tiene usted la botella/caja?

¿Ha vomitado?

¿Le dio algún tratamiento?
¿El carbón?
¿Ipecacuana?
¿Cómo ha estado comportándose desde entonces?

11. Trauma: Falls

Did he/she/you fall? How?

How far did he/she/you fall?

What did he/she/you land on?
On what part of the body did he/she/you fall?
Did he/she/you hit his/her/your head?

Was he/she/you wearing a helmet?
Did he/she/you lose consciousness?
For how long?

Did he/she/you cry right away after the accident?

Has he/she/you seemed confused, sleepy, dizzy, weak?

Has he/she/you vomited since the accident?

Does anything (else) hurt?

Is he/she/you immunized against tetanus?

11. Traumatismo: Caidas

¿Se cayó?
¿Cómo?

¿De qué altura cayó?

¿Adonde se cayó?
¿Sobre qué parte de su cuerpo cayó?
¿Se golpeó la cabeza?

¿Estaba con casco?
¿Perdió la consciencia?
¿Por cuánto tiempo?

¿Lloró inmediatamente después del accidente?

¿Ha parecido confundido/a, cansado/a, mareado/a, débil?

¿Ha vomitado desde el accidente?

¿Le [to child: te] duele algo más?

¿Está vacunado/a contra el tétanos?

11. Trauma: Falls (continued)

When was his/her/your last tetanus shot?

We will need to do some X-rays.

This cut will need a few stitches.

11. Traumatismo: Caidas (continuación)

¿Cuándo recibio su última vacuna contra el tétanos?

Tenemos que hacer algunas radiografías.

Esta cortadura necesitará algunos puntos.

12. Trauma: Motor Vehicle Accident (MVA)

(See questions regarding head injury in Section 11 on p. 165)

Was he/she/you in a car accident?
What happened?
When?

How fast was the car going?
Where was the impact on the car _____?
(Front, right/left side, back?)

Where (in which seat) was he/she/you?
Was he/she in a car seat?

12. Traumatismo: Accidente en Vehiculo Motorizado

¿Tuvo un accidente de automóvil?
¿Qué pasó?
¿Cuándo?

¿A qué velocidad venía el carro?
¿En qué parte del carro fué el impacto _____?
(Adelante, en el lado derecho/izquierdo, atrás?)

¿Dónde (en qué asiento) estaba?
¿Estaba él/ella en una silla para niños?

Was he/she/you wearing a seat belt?	¿Estaba usando un cinturón de seguridad?
How much damage was done to the car?	¿Cuánto daño sufrió el carro?
Did the windshield break?	¿Se quebró el parabrisas?

13. Trauma: Musculoskeletal

13. Traumatismo: Musculoesquelético

How did this happen? When? Show me how you did it.	¿Como pasó el accidente? ¿Cuándo? Enséñeme como ocurrió.
Show me where it hurts.	Muéstrame donde duele.
Did he/she/you hit his/her/your head?	¿Se golpeó en la cabeza?
Did he/she/you hurt anything else?	¿Se golpeó en alguna otra parte?
Does it hurt when I squeeze here, or move it this way?	¿Duele cuando aprieto aquí, o lo muevo de esta manera?
Has this happened before? When? How many times?	¿Ha sufrido el mismo accidente antes? ¿Cuándo? ¿Cuántas veces?

Description of Pain	**Descripción del Dolor**
Has he/she/you been having pain?	¿Ha estado teniendo dolor?
Are you in pain now?	¿Tienes dolor ahora?
Where is the pain? Show me with one finger.	¿Dónde está el dolor? Muéstrame con el dedo.
Does the pain go anywhere?	¿Se va el dolor para algún lado?
What is the pain like?	¿Cómo es el dolor?
Is the pain:	¿Es el dolor:
mild?	leve?
moderate?	moderado?
severe?	severo?
constant?	constante?
sharp, like a knife?	agudo, como de un cuchillo?
dull and aching?	sordo?
like pressure?	como presión?
burning?	ardiente?
gassy?	como gas?
crampy?	como calambre?
shooting/pricking?	punzante?
throbbing?	pulsátil?
Does it come and go?	¿Va y viene?
When did the pain first start?	¿Cuándo empezó el dolor?
Did the pain start gradually or suddenly?	¿Empezó gradualmente o repentinamente?
Has the pain changed?	¿Ha cambiado el dolor?
Is the pain worse, better, or the same as before?	¿Está el dolor peor, mejor, o igual que antes?

How often does he/she/you have the pain?	¿Con qué frecuencia tiene el dolor?
All the time (without interruption)?	¿Todo el tiempo (sin interrupción)?
How many times per day, per week, per month?	¿Cuántas veces al día, a la semana, al mes?
How long does the pain last?	¿Cuánto dura el dolor?
Does anything make the pain better?	¿Hay algo que alivie el dolor?
Worse?	¿Qué lo empeora?
What brings on the pain?	¿Qué ocasiona el dolor?
food? Which ones?	comida? ¿Cuáles?
How long after eating does the pain begin?	¿Cuánto tiempo después de comer empieza el dolor?
an empty stomach?	el estómago vacío?
bowel movements?	las evacuaciones?
urination?	el orinar?
a particular movement? Show me.	un movimiento en particular? Muéstrame.
exercise?	ejercicio?
(emotional) stress?	tensión (emocional)?
Do other symptoms come along with the pain?	¿Hay otros síntomas que acompañan el dolor?
Does the pain wake him/her/you up at night?	¿El dolor lo/la despierta en la noche?
Does he/she cry because of the pain?	¿Llora del dolor?
Has he/she/you taken anything for the pain?	¿Ha tomado alguna medicina para el dolor?
What? When?	¿Qué? ¿Cuándo?
Did it help?	¿Le ayudó?

Examination Instructions	Instrucciones Para el Examen
Please take off all his/her/your clothes except for underwear/diaper.	Por favor, quítese la ropa excepto su ropa interior/pañal.
Here is an examination gown to wear.	Aquí hay una bata para que se ponga.
Please take off his/her/your:	Por favor quítese:
shirt	la camisa
pants	los pantalones
shoes and socks	zapatos y calcetines
underwear	la ropa interior
Please hold him in your arms for now.	Sosténgalo/la en sus brazos por ahora.
Hold (his/her arms, legs, head) like this.	Sostenga (sus brazos, sus piernas, su cabeza) así.
Put him/her on the examining table.	Póngalo/la sobre la camilla.
	(Note: the following are in the familiar "tu" form.)
Please sit over here.	Siéntate aquí, por favor.
Please	Por favor
lie down	acuéstate
sit up	siéntate
stand up	párate
turn over, around	voltéate
bend over and touch your toes	agáchate y toca la punta de tus pies
walk that way	camina hacia allá

now walk toward me	ahora camina hacia mí
stand on your (left, right) foot	párate en tu pie (izquierdo, derecho)
do this	haz esto
look at this	mira esto

Watch my finger with your eyes.

Mira mi dedo con tus ojos.

Don't turn your head.

No voltees la cabeza.

Open your mouth and say aah.

Abre la boca y di aah.

Stick out your tongue.

Saca la lengua.

Breathe deeply (with your mouth open).

Respira profundo (con la boca abierta).

Hold your breath for a moment.

Contén tu respiración por un momento.

Relax your stomach. How ticklish you are!

Relaja el estómago. ¡Qué cosquillas tienes!

Does anything hurt? Show me with your finger.

¿Te duele algo? Muéstrame con el dedo.

Does this hurt? Tell me what hurts.

¿Te duele esto? Dime lo que te duele.

Discharge Instructions

1. Medication
2. General Instructions
3. Fever
4. Gastrointestinal
5. Respiratory
6. Neurology
7. Dermatology
8. Musculoskeletal Trauma

Instrucciones de Alta

(Words often used in following section are provided here; for additional words, see pp. 197-208.)

one	uno/a
two	dos
three	tres
four	cuatro
five	cinco
six	seis
as needed	como sea necesario

1. Medication

Take _____ pills
_____ times per day.
(tablets, teaspoons, tablespoons, dropperfuls)

Place _____ drops in
  each ear
  each eye
  right ear
  right eye
  left ear
  left eye
  _____ times per day.

1. Medicación

Tome _____ pastillas
_____ veces al día.
(tabletas, cucharaditas, cucharadas, goteros)

Póngale _____ gotas en
  cada oído
  cada ojo
  el oído derecho
  el ojo derecho
  el oído izquierdo
  el ojo izquierdo
  _____ veces al día.

172

Place the ointment:	Póngale el ungüento:
in each eye.	en cada ojo.
the right eye.	el ojo derecho.
the left eye.	el ojo izquierdo.
_____ times per day.	_____ veces al día.
Apply the cream (ointment) _____ times per day.	Póngale la crema (el ungüento) _____ veces al día.
Take _____ puffs/ inhalations _____ times per day.	Tome _____ inhalaciones _____ veces al día.
Place _____cc of _____ into _____ cc of (normal saline) in the nebulizer (machine).	Póngale _____ cc de _____ en _____cc de (agua salina) en la nebulizador (máquina).
Your child should receive _____ nebulizer treatments per day.	Su niño/a debe recibir _____ tratamientos con el nebulizador al día.
Give your child the medication only when you feel he/she needs it.	Dele a su niño/a la medicina solamente cuando usted crea que él/ella la necesita.

2. General Instructions

Go to the nearest emergency department now.

Observe your child carefully.

Some danger signs are if your baby:

  becomes lethargic/tired

  cries a lot

  plays less

  does not eat well

If your child gets worse:

  Bring him/her to the emergency department.

  Return immediately.

Call the clinic if your child is not improving. Return (tomorrow, in _____days, weeks, months).

I would like to see your child again in _____ (days, weeks, months, years).

Here is an appointment for _____.

2. Instrucciones Generales

Vaya al servicio de urgencias cercana ahora.

Observe a su niño/a con atención.

Son señas de peligro si su niño/a:

  se pone letárgico/a o muy cansado/a

  llora mucho

  juega menos

  no come bien

Si se empeora su niño/a:

  Traiga él/su al servicio de urgencias.

  Regresen inmediatamente.

Llame a la clínica si su niño/a, no está mejorando. Regresen (mañana; en _____ días, semanas, meses).

Quiero ver a su niño/a otra vez en _____ (días, semanas, meses, años).

Aquí tiene una cita para _____.

3. Fever

Take your child's temperature (every _____ hours, _____ times a day).

To take your child's temperature, place the thermometer in his/her (mouth, rectum, armpit) for 3 to 5 minutes.

Please call me (return to the clinic) if his/her temperature is greater than _____ degrees Celsius/Fahrenheit.

To help your child's fever go down, dress him/her in light clothing. You may also bathe him/her in lukewarm water for 15 to 20 minutes.
Take him/her out if he/she begins to shiver.

Give your child lots of fluid to drink.

3. Fiebre

Tómele la temperatura (cada _____ horas, _____ veces al día).

Para tomar la temperatura, póngale el termómetro en su (boca, recto, axila) por tres a cinco minutos.

Llámeme (regresen a la clínica) si su temperatura es más de _____ grados Celsius/Fahrenheit.

Para bajar la temperatura, debe vestirle con ropa ligera. También puede bañarlo/la en agua tibia por quince a veinte minutos. Si comienza él/ella a tiritar, sáquelo/la del baño.

Déle a su niño/a mucho líquido para tomar.

4. Gastrointestinal

Try to give your child _____ (tablespoons, ounces, cups) of _____ (oral rehydration solution) every _____ hours for _____ days.

You can use a (spoon, dropper, syringe).

Give your child (regular formula, milk, juice) half diluted with water for _____ hours/days.

Do not give your child milk or dairy products for _____ days.

Foods which may help your child's diarrhea/constipation are:

Diarrhea

rice cereal

rice

potatoes (not fried)

noodles

crackers

toast

bananas

4. Gastrointestinal

Trate de darle a su niño/a _____ (cucharas, onzas, tazas) de _____ (suero) cada _____ horas por _____ días.

Puede usar (una cuchara, un gotero, una jeringa).

Déle a su niño/a (fórmula, leche, jugo) diluido a la mitad con agua por _____ horas/días.

No le de leche o productos lácteos por _____ días.

Comidas que pueden mejorar la diarrea/el estreñamiento son:

Diarrea

cereal de arroz

arroz

papas (no fritas)

fideos

galletas saltinas

pan tostado

bananas

Constipation	**Estreñimiento**
fruit juices	jugos de fruta
apricot juice	jugo de durazno
apple juice	jugo de manzana
prune juice	jugo de pruna/ ciruela seca
bran cereal	cereal con fibra
bran muffins	panecillos (muffins) con fibra
whole wheat bread	pan integral
applesauce	puré de manzana

5. Respiratory

    Some danger signs are:

        increased difficulty breathing

        pale or blue lip/skin color

        decreased eating or drinking

        problems taking the bottle

        faster breathing

        unusual drowsiness or fussiness

Place a humidifier in your child's bedroom.

5. Respiratorio

    Señas de peligro son:

        más dificultad para respirar

        labios o piel de color pálido o azul

        disminución en lo que come o bebe

        problemas tomando la botella

        respiraciones más rápidas

        cansancio o irritibilidad

Ponga un humedificador en el dormitorio de su niño/a.

5. Respiratory (continued)

If your child has trouble breathing:

> have him/her sit in the bathroom to breathe in the steam of a hot shower.

> try taking him/her outside into the night air.

6. Neurology

Some danger signs are:

> vomiting

> dizziness

> worsening headache

> unsteadiness while walking

> weakness of the arms or legs

> abnormal sleepiness

> confusion

> difficulty speaking

If he/she shows any of these signs, call the clinic (bring him/her to the emergency department).

5. Respiratorio (continuación)

Si su niño/a tiene dificultad para respirar:

> llévelo/la al cuarto de baño para respirar el vapor de una ducha caliente.

> pruebe sacándolo/la al aire de la noche.

6. Neurológico

Algunas señas de peligro son:

> vómitos

> mareos

> dolor de cabeza que empeora

> inestabilidad cuando camina

> debilidad en los brazos o piernas

> cansancio más que lo normal

> confusión

> dificultad para hablar

Si muestra él/ella alguna de estas señas, llame a la clínica (traiga él/su al servicio de urgencias).

7. Dermatology

To decrease the itching, you may give your child a bath in lukewarm water (with _____).

You should soak the _____ in warm water for _____ minutes _____ times per day.

Apply the cream (ointment) _____ times per day.

8. Musculoskeletal Trauma

Apply ice (a warm compress) for _____ minutes _____ times per day (before/after exercise).

He/she/you should rest (this, the _____) for _____ days.

You will need to use (crutches, an Ace bandage, a sling, a cast) for _____ (days, weeks).

He/she/you should elevate his/her/your _____ (hand, arm, foot, leg).

7. Dermatologia

Para que no pique tanto, puede darle a su niño/a un baño con agua tibia (con _____).

Debe remojar el/la _____ en agua caliente por _____ minutos _____ veces al día.

Póngale la crema (el ungüento) _____ veces al día.

8. Traumatismo Musculoesquelético

Aplique hielo (una compresa cálida) por _____ minutos _____ veces al día (antes/después del ejercicio).

Debe descansar (esto, el/la _____) por _____ días.

Vas a tener que usar (muletas, un vendaje "Ace," un cabestrillo, un yeso) por _____ (dias, semanas).

Debe elevar su _____ (mano, brazo, pie, pierna).

179

Special Issues

Abuse Screening Questions

(Note: It is particularly important to obtain appropriate translation and expertise when abuse is suspected. The questions provided here should only be used when absolutely necessary and no alternatives are available. They are not adequate for evaluation.)

◆ **To parent:**

What happened?

With whom does your child spend time alone?

Is there any chance your child could have been hurt by someone? By whom?

Is there any possibility that your child could have been abused (sexually abused)?

By whom?

◆ **To child:**

What happened?

Show me what happened.

Has anyone hurt you?

Has anyone touched you in places you don't like?

◆ **Al padre/madre:**

¿Qué pasó?

¿Con quién se queda su niño/a a solas?

¿Hay alguna posibilidad de que alguien le haya hecho daño? ¿Quién?

¿Hay alguna posibilidad de que su niño/a haya sido maltratado/a (maltratado/a sexualmente)?

¿Por quién?

◆ **Al niño:**

¿Qué pasó?

Enséñame que pasó.

¿Alguien te ha hecho daño?

¿Alguna persona te ha tocado en lugares que no te gusta?

Has anyone touched you under your clothes?

¿Alguna persona te ha tocado adentro de tu ropa?

Do you ever feel frightened?

¿Alguna vez te has sentido asustado/a?

What makes you feel scared?

¿Que te hace sentir miedo?

What happens when _____ is angry?

¿Qué pasa cuando _____ está enojado/a?

It is very important to talk more about this.

Es muy importante hablar más sobre esto.

Please wait while I get a translator/social worker/psychiatrist/ psychologist/nurse.

Por favor, espere mientras busco un traductor/trabajador/a social/psiquiatra/ psicólogo/enfermero/a.

Ancillary Services	**Servicios de Apoyo**
◆ **Registration**	◆ **Registración**
What is his/her/your name?	¿Cuál es su nombre?
last name?	¿apellido?
first name?	¿nombre?
middle initial?	¿inicial de su segundo nombre?
middle name?	¿segundo nombre?
What is his/her/your birth date?	¿Cuál es su fecha de nacimiento?
What is his/her/your social security number?	¿Cuál es su número de seguro social?
Do you have a driver's license or picture ID?	¿Tiene usted una licencia de conducir o identificación con foto?
What is his/her/your address?	¿Cuál es su dirección?
Is there an apartment number?	¿Tiene número de apartamento?
city?	¿ciudad?
state?	¿estado?
zip code?	¿código postal?
telephone number?	¿número de teléfono?
at home?	¿en la casa?
at work?	¿en el trabajo?
What is his/her/your father's name?	¿Cómo se llama su padre?
address?	¿dirección?
phone number?	¿teléfono?

What is his/her/your mother's name?	¿Cómo se llama su madre?
mother's maiden name?	¿el apellido de soltera?
address?	¿dirección?
phone number?	¿teléfono?
What is your relationship to the patient?	¿Cuál es su relación con el paciente?
In case of emergency, who should be contacted?	¿En caso de emergencia, quién debe ser contactado?
What is their name?	¿Cuál es el nombre?
relationship?	¿relación?
address?	¿dirección?
telephone?	¿teléfono?
Who is the guardian?	¿Quién es el apoderado?
What is his/her/your marital status?	¿Cuál es su estado civil?
What is his/her/your race?	¿Cuál es su raza?
What is his/her/your religion?	¿Cuál es su religión?
What language does he/she/you speak?	¿Qué idioma habla?
Does he/she/you have medical insurance? What type?	¿Tiene seguro médico? ¿De que tipo?
Do you have the insurance card?	¿Tiene la tarjeta del seguro?
Who is the policy holder?	¿Quién es el asegurado?

◆ Registration
(continued)

Who should receive
the bill?

What is the address
and zip code of this
person?

Does either parent have
a job? What type?

What is the name
and address of the
employer? Phone?

Would you like to apply
for financial aid?
Free care?

Who is his/her/your
regular doctor?

He/she/you should
return here again
in _____ (days, weeks,
months, years).

What day/time is good
for you?

You have an
appointment for _____.

Is this date and time
good for you?

Here is an appointment
card with the date.

◆ Registro
(continuación)

¿Quién debe recibir
la cuenta?

¿Cuál es la dirección
y código postal de esa
persona?

¿Trabaja alguno de
los padres? ¿En qué?

¿Cuál es el nombre
y dirección del
empleador? ¿Teléfono?

¿Piensa solicitar
ayuda financiera?
¿Cuidado gratis?

¿Quién es su médico
regular?

Él/ella/usted debe
regresar en _____
(días, semanas,
meses, años).

¿Que día/hora es
mejor para usted?

Usted tiene una cita
para _____.

¿Es éste día y hora
conveniente para
usted?

Acá tiene una tarjeta
con la fecha y hora de
la cita.

184

◆ Radiology

I am going to take an X-ray of his/her/your:

    chest

    abdomen

    arm

    hand

    foot

    leg

    head

    neck

    back

Is there any possibility that you are pregnant?

X-rays can be harmful to your baby if you are pregnant.

Someone else must hold your baby (child).

Please take off:
    all of his/her/your clothes
    clothes from the waist up
    jewelry
    bra

◆ Radiología

Le voy a tomar a él/ella/usted una radiografía del:

    tórax

    abdomen

    brazo

    mano

    pie

    pierna

    cabeza

    cuello

    espalda

¿Hay alguna posibilidad que usted esté embarazada?

Si usted está embarazada los rayos X pueden hacerle daño a su bebé.

Alguna otra persona deberá sostener a su bebé (niño).

Por favor, quítese(le):
    toda la ropa

    la ropa de la cintura para arriba
    las joyas
    el sostén (brassiere)

◆ **Radiology**
  (continued)

Please put on the gown
so that it opens in the
front/back.

Do not move.

Hold your child like this.

Hold him/her still.

He/she/you must be
held in the light.

Roll onto your side and
face that wall.

Take a deep breath
and hold it.

Please sit down here
and wait for a few
minutes.

Do not get dressed until
we check the films.

We may need to take
some more films.

We are all finished.

You may go now.

Return to your doctor.

Return to the
emergency
department.

◆ **Radiologia**
  (continuación)

Por favor, póngase
el mandil con la abertura
para adelante/atrás.

No se mueva.

Agarre al niño/la
niña así.

Manténgalo/a quieto.

Manténgalo/a en
la luz.

Voltéese sobre su
lado y mire a la pared.

Respire profundamente
y retenga el aire.

Por favor, siéntesé
aquí y espere algunos
minutos.

No se ponga la ropa
hasta que examinemos
las radiografías.

Es posible que
necesitemos tomar
más radiografías.

Hemos terminado.

Puede salir ahora.

Puede regresar a la
oficina del doctor.

Vuelta al servicio
de urgencias.

◆ **Ultrasound**

Drink _____ cups of water.

Do not urinate until after the test.

I am going to use a gel which will feel cold (warm).

This will not hurt.

◆ **MRI/CT**

Can he/she/you lie still for _____ minutes?

We will be giving your child some medicine so that he/she will sleep during the test.

Does he/she/you have any metal or surgical appliances in his/her/ your body?

Does he/she/you have claustrophobia?

◆ **Ultrasonido (Sonograma)**

Beba (tome) _____ vasos de agua.

No orine hasta que termine la prueba.

Voy a usar un gel que se siente frío (tibio).

Esto no va a doler.

◆ **Resonancia magnética/tomografía**

¿Podrá él/ella/usted estarse quieto por _____ minutos?

Le vamos a dar una medicina a su niño para que duerma durante la prueba.

¿Tiene él/ella/usted algún material metálico o quirúrgico en su cuerpo?

¿Sufre él/ella/usted de claustrofobia (temor a sitios cerrados)?

◆ **Laboratory**

Do you understand English?

May I please see your papers?

Please sit in the chair on the left, right.

I am going to take blood from his/her/your:

    arm

    finger

    heel

    toe

I am going to use this finger.

Please hold your child like this.

Please hold his/her elbow. I will hold the wrist.

Please do not move.

Please hold your child still.

Please roll up your (right, left) sleeve.

Close your hand.

You may open your hand now.

◆ **Laboratorio**

¿Entiende inglés?

¿Podría ver sus papeles/ documentos/formas?

Por favor, siéntese en la silla de la izquierda, derecha.

Voy a tomar una muestra de sangre del:

    brazo

    dedo

    talón

    dedo del pie

Voy a usar este dedo.

Por favor, agarre así a su niño/a.

Por favor, agárrele el codo. Yo agarraré la muñeca.

Por favor, no se mueva.

Por favor, mantenga quieto a su niño.

Por favor, súbase la manga (derecha, izquierda).

Cierre la mano.

Puede abrir la mano ahora.

Please press here with your fingers.	Por favor, apriete aquí con sus dedos.
How do you feel?	¿Cómo se siente?
Do you feel dizzy?	¿Se siente mareado/a?
Please put your head down.	Por favor, baje la cabeza.
Sometimes we need to try more than one time.	A veces tenemos que tratar más de una vez.
We will need to try again.	Debemos tratar nuevamente.
The bathroom is here.	El baño queda aquí.
Please urinate into the cup.	Por favor, orine en el vaso (recipiente).
First clean with the towelettes from front to back.	Primero límpiese con las toallitas de adelante para atrás.
Then urinate into the cup.	Luego orine en el vaso.
We would like the urine in the middle of your stream.	Necesitamos una muestra de la mitad del chorro.
We need a stool sample.	Necesitamos una muestra de las heces.
Please collect it into this cup, and bring it back here:	Por favor colecte la muestra en este recipiente y tráigala:
as soon as possible	lo antes posible
tomorrow	mañana
next week	la próxima semana
any time the laboratory is open	cuando el laboratorio esté abierto

◆ Laboratory (continued)

Are you fasting?

Please drink all of this in 10 minutes.

Your doctor will have the results in 1 (hour, day, week, month).

◆ EKG

We are going to test his/her/your heart.

Do not be afraid.

This will not hurt.

Take off everything from the waist up.

- bra
- shirt
- pants
- panty hose
- tights

Please put on the gown so that it opens in the front/back.

Please have a seat in the chair.

Please lay down here.

I will be back in a few minutes.

◆ Laboratorio (continuación)

¿Está usted en ayunas?

Por favor, bébase todo esto en los próximos diez minutos.

Su doctor tendrá los resultados en un(a) (hora, día, semana, mes).

◆ Electrocardiograma

Vamos a hacer una prueba de su corazón.

No tenga temor (miedo).

Esto no va a doler.

Quítese todo de la cintura para arriba.

- el sostén (brassiere)
- la camisa
- los pantalones
- mallas (truza)
- calcetines

Por favor, póngase el mandil con la abertura para adelante/atrás.

Por favor, siéntese en la silla.

Por favor, acuéstese aquí.

Regresaré en breves minutos.

Please lie still.

Por favor, quédese quieto.

Please take this back to your doctor.

Por favor, lléve esto a su doctor.

Please return now to:

Por favor, regrese ahora:

   your doctor's office

   a la oficina del doctor

   the emergency department

   el servicio de urgencias

Developmental Milestones — Gross Motor

Motor Grueso

Age	Can he/she:	¿Puede su niño/a:
1 mo	lift head while lying on stomach?	levantar la cabeza mientras está acostado/a boca abajo?
2 mos	hold head steady while sitting upright?	sostener firme la cabeza cuando está sentado/a?
3 mos	support self on legs with help?	sostenerse en las piernas con ayuda?
4 mos	roll over?	darse vuelta?
6 mos	sit without support?	sentarse sin ayuda?
7-8 mos	stand holding on to things?	pararse agarrándose de las cosas?
11 mos	stand alone?	pararse solo/a?
11 mos	walk holding on?	caminar agarrándose de las cosas?
13-14 mos	walk well?	caminar bien?
14-20 mos	run?	correr?
18-22 mos	walk up steps?	subir gradas o escalones?
1 1/2-2 yrs	kick a ball?	patear un balón?
2-4 yrs	jump?	saltar?
2 1/2 yrs	balance on each foot?	balancearse en un pie?
3-4 yrs	hop?	brincar en un pie?
4-5 yrs	heel-to-toe walk (like this)?	andar del talón a la punta de los pies (como por ejemplo)?

Developmental Milestones — Visual Motor

Age	Can he/she:	Motor Visual ¿Puede su niño/a:
1-3 mos	visually follow past midline?	seguir visualmente de un lado al otro?
3-4 mos	grasp toy?	agarrar un juguete?
4-5 mos	reach out toward objects?	tender la mano hacia cosas?
9 mos	grasp with thumb and finger?	agarrar con el pulgar y un dedo (hacer una pinza)?
12-15 mos	drink from cup?	tomar de una taza?
12-15 mos	scribble?	hacer garabatos?
18 mos	feed self using spoon?	comer con cuchara?
18-20 mos	undress self?	desvestirse solo/a?
3-4 yrs	copy circle? *(to child: draw this)*	copiar círculos? *(dibuja esto)*
3-4 yrs	dress self with supervision?	vestirse con supervisión?
3-4 yrs	draw a person with 3 parts?	dibujar una persona con tres partes?

Developmental Milestones — Language

Lenguaje

Age	Can he/she:	¿Puede su niño/a:
1-3 mos	coo?	hacer "agus"?
4-5 mos	orient to voice?	responder a la voz?
6-9 mos	babble?	balbucear?
9-11 mos	say dada or mama (meaning you)?	decir papá o mamá (refiriendose a usted)?
11-13 mos	say one word?	decir una palabra?
15 mos	say three to six words?	decir de tres a seis palabras?
2 yrs	make a two-word phrase?	hacer una frase de dos palabras?
2 yrs	know six body parts?	saber seis partes del cuerpo?
2-3 yrs	follow simple instructions?	seguir instrucciones simples?
3 yrs	speak understandably? (Do you understand all that he/she says?)	hablar claramente? (¿Entiende usted todo lo que le dice?)

194

Developmental Milestones — Social Development

Desarrollo Social

Age	Can he/she:	¿Puede su niño/a:
0-2 mos	smile (spontaneously)?	sonreír (espontáneamente)?
1 mos	smile when you play with him/her?	sonreír cuando juega usted con él/ella?
2-3 mos	laugh?	reírse?
8 mos	wave bye-bye?	decir adiós con la mano?
9 mos	indicate wants?	indicar lo que quiere?
1-2 yrs	imitate activities?	imitar actividades?
2 yrs	wash and dry hands?	lavarse y secarse las manos?
2 yrs	put on any clothing?	ponerse alguna ropa?
2 1/2 yrs	say first and last name?	decir su nombre y apellido?
3 yrs	name friend?	nombrar un amigo?
3-4 yrs	play games in groups?	jugar en grupos?

Lead Toxicity Screening Questions

Do you know if there is lead paint in your home?

Does your child have a brother or sister or friend who has had lead poisoning?

Think about your home, homes of relatives or babysitters, and day care centers. Do any of these buildings have lead?

Does your child spend time in these types of buildings?

Buildings with peeling or chipping paint?

Buildings that have been recently remodeled or are being remodeled now?

Was this building built before 1950?

Do any adults that your child has contact with work with lead, such as construction, welding, or pottery?

Do you live near any factories?

What type of factory?

Preguntas de Despistaje de Intoxicacion por Plomo

¿Sabe si hay pintura con plomo en su casa?

¿Tiene el niño algún hermano/a o amigo que se halla intoxicado con plomo?

Piense acerca de su casa, casa de parientes, niñeras y guardería. ¿Alguna de estos edificios tiene plomo?

¿Pasa tiempo su niño en estos lugares?

¿Donde la pintura se está pelando (descascarando)?

¿Que han sido recientemente remodelados o están siendo remodelados?

¿Fué este edificio construído antes de mil novecientos sesenta?

¿Hay algún adulto con el que el niño mantenga contacto que trabaje con plomo, como por ejemplo en construcción, soldadura, o cerámica?

¿Vive usted cerca a alguna fabrica?

¿Que tipo de fabrica?

Additional Words and Phrases

1. Questions
2. Terms of Relation
3. Time
4. Numbers
5. Anatomy

1. Questions

who	quién
what	qué
where	dónde
when	cuándo
why	por qué
how	cómo
to where	adónde
since when	desde cuándo
how long ago	hace cuánto tiempo
how often	con qué frecuencia
how much	cuánto
at what time	a qué hora
at what age	a qué edad

2. Terms of Relation

worse than	peor que
better than	mejor que
the same (as)	lo mismo (que)
more than	más que
less than	menos que
after	después
before	antes
during	mientras
bigger	más grande
smaller	más pequeño
next to	al lado de

3. Time

second	segundo
minute	minuto
hour	hora
day	día
week	semana
month	mes

year	año
morning	mañana
afternoon	tarde
night	noche
tomorrow	mañana
yesterday	ayer
spring	primavera
summer	verano
fall	otoño
winter	invierno
Monday	lunes
Tuesday	martes
Wednesday	miércoles
Thursday	jueves
Friday	viernes
Saturday	sábado
Sunday	domingo
January	enero
February	febrero
March	marzo
April	abril
May	mayo
June	junio
July	julio
August	agosto
September	septiembre
October	octubre
November	noviembre
December	diciembre

4. Numbers

1	uno
2	dos
3	tres
4	cuatro
5	cinco
6	seis
7	siete
8	ocho
9	nueve
10	diez
11	once

```
12 ............................ doce
13 ............................ trece
14 ............................ catorce
15 ............................ quince
16 ............................ dieciséis
17 ............................ diecisiete
18 ............................ dieciocho
19 ............................ diecinueve
20 ............................ veinte
50 ............................ cincuenta
100 .......................... cien
1000 ........................ mil
```

5. Anatomy

```
abdomen .................. el abdomen
ankle ....................... el tobillo
anus ........................ el ano
appendix .................. el apéndice
arch (of foot) ............ el arco (del pie)
arm .......................... el brazo
armpit ...................... la axila
artery ...................... la arteria
back ........................ la espalda
"belly" ..................... el abdomen, el vientre
"belly button" ............ el ombligo
bladder .................... la vejiga
blood ....................... la sangre
body ........................ el cuerpo
bone ........................ el hueso
bone marrow ............. médula del hueso
brain ........................ el cerebro
breast ...................... el pecho
buttocks ................... las nalgas
calf .......................... la pantorilla
cervix ...................... el cérvix, el cuello de la matriz
cheek ....................... la mejilla
chest ....................... el pecho, el tórax
chin ......................... la barbilla
clavicle .................... la clavícula
clitoris ..................... el clítoris
diaphragm ................ el diafragma
ear (external) ........... la oreja
```

ear (internal)	el oído
elbow	el codo
embryo	el embrión
esophagus	el esófago
eye	el ojo
eyebrow	la ceja
eyelash	la pestaña
eyelid	el párpado
face	la cara
fallopian tubes	los tubos (trompas de Falopio)
finger	el dedo
fontanelle	la mollera, la fontanela
foot	el pie
forearm	el antebrazo
forehead	la frente
foreskin	el prepucio
gall bladder	la vesícula biliar
gland	la glándula
gums	las encias
hair	el pelo
hand	la mano
head	la cabeza
heart	el corazón
hip	la cadera
hymen	el himen
intestine	los intestinos
– large intestine	el intestino grueso
– small intestine	el intestino delgado
iris	el iris
jaw	la mandíbula
joint	la articulación
kidney	el riñón
knee	la rodilla
knuckle	el nudillo
leg	la pierna
ligament	el ligamento
lips	los labios
liver	el hígado
lungs	los pulmones
lymph node	el ganglio

mouth	la boca
muscle	el músculo
nail	la uña
nape of neck	la nuca
navel	el ombligo
neck	el cuello
nerve	el nervio
nipple	el pezón
nose	la nariz
organ	el órgano
ovary	el ovario
pancreas	el páncreas
penis	el pene
prostate	la próstata
pupil	la pupila
rectum	el recto
rib	la costilla
scalp	el cuero cabelludo
scrotum	el escroto
shoulder	el hombro
skeleton	el esquéleto
skin	la piel
skull	el cráneo
spinal cord	médula espinal
spine	la columna vertebral
spleen	el bazo
stomach	el estómago
tendon	el tendón
testicle	el testículo
throat	la garganta
thumb	el pulgar
thymus	el timo
thyroid	la tiroides
toe	el dedo del pie
tongue	la lengua
tonsils	las amígdalas
tooth	el diente
urethra	uretra
uterus	el útero, la matriz
vagina	la vagina
vein	la vena

vessel	el vaso
vocal cords	las cuerdas vocales
womb	la matriz, vientre materno
wrist	la muñeca

6. Body products

bile	la bilis
blood	la sangre
breast milk	la leche del pecho
discharge	el flujo, secreción
hormone	la hormona
menstrual flow	el flujo menstrual
mucus	el moco
phlegm	la flema
pus	la pus
saliva	la saliva
a sample	una muestra
semen	el semen
sputum	el esputo
stool	el popó, las heces, la evacuación
tears	las lágrimas
a test	una prueba
urine	la orina
vomit	el vómito

7. Pathology

abscess	el absceso
acne	el acné
AIDS	SIDA (síndrome de inmunodeficiencia adquirida)
allergy	alergia
anemia	la anemia
appendicitis	apendicitis
arthritis	la artritis
asthma	el asma
athlete's foot	pie de atleta
bacterium	la bacteria
blind	ciego/a
blood clot	el coágulo
a blow	un golpe
broken bone	la fractura

202

bronchitis	la bronquitis
bruise	el moretón
burn	la quemadura
cancer	el cáncer
CHF	fallo cardíaco
chicken pox	la varicela
cholera	el cólera
cold	el resfrío
concussion	concusión
confusion	confusión
constipation	el estreñimiento
cough	la tos
cut	cortadura
deaf	sordo/a
dehydration	deshidratación
depression	la depresión
dermatitis	la dermatitis
diabetes	la diabetes
diarrhea	la diarrea
diphtheria	la difteria
dizziness	mareos
ear infection	infección de oído
eczema	el eczema
epilepsy	la epilepsia
fever	la fiebre
flu	la gripe
fracture	la fractura
hay fever	fiebre del heno
fungus	el hongo
gallstone	el cálculo biliar
gastritis	la gastritis
headache	dolor de cabeza, cefalea
hemophilia	hemofilia
hemorrhage	la hemorragia
hepatitis	la hepatitis, inflamación del hígado
hernia	la hernia
herpes	herpes
hypertension	presión alta
illness	la enfermedad
infection	infección

inflammation	inflamación
IBD	enfermedad inflamatoria del intestino
influenza	la gripe, influenza
injury	la herida
laryngitis	la laringitis
leukemia	la leucemia
lice	los piojos
lymphoma	el linfoma
malaria	malaria, paludismo
malnutrition	desnutrición
measles	el sarampión
meningitis	la meningitis
mononucleosis	mononucleosis
mumps	las paperas
murmur	soplo cardíaco
nausea	la náusea
nightmare	la pesadilla
numbness	adormecimiento
obesity	la obesidad
pain	el dolor
parasite	el parásito
pertussis	la tos convulsiva o ferina
pneumonia	la neumonía, pulmonía
polio	parálisis infantil, polio
protein	la proteína
psoriasis	psoriasis
rash	la erupción
rubella	rubéola, sarampión alemán
scrape	la raspadura
seizure	el ataque, la convulsión
sexual abuse	abuso sexual
shock	el choque
sinusitis	la sinusitis
sore	la llaga
sore throat	dolor de garganta
sprain	el esguince, torcedura
stone	el cálculo
strabismus	bizco, estrabismo
strain	tensión
strep throat	amigdalitis por estreptococo

stroke	derrame cerebral
swelling	la hinchazón
syphilis	la sífilis
tetanus	el tétanos
thrush	afta
tuberculosis	la tuberculosis
tumor	el tumor
ulcer	la úlcera
unconscious	pérdida de consciencia
venereal disease	enfemedad venérea
virus	el virus
worms	las lombrices
wound	la herida

8. Therapy

anesthetic	el anestésico
antacid	el antiácido
antibiotic	el antibiótico
anticoagulant	el anticoagulante
bandage	el vendaje
"band aid"	la curita
bath	el baño
brace	el braguero
braces (teeth)	los frenos
calcium	el calcio
cane	el caño, bastón
capsule	la cápsula
cast	el yeso
cathartic	el purgante
catheter	el catéter
chemotherapy	la quimioterápia
compress	la compresa
contact lens	el lente de contacto
cream	la crema
crutch	la muleta
decongestant	el descongestionante
dental floss	hilo dental
dialysis	diálisis
diaphragm	el diafrágma
drop	la gota
droppers	el gotero
drug	la droga (street drugs)

emetic	emético
enema	el enema
fluoride	el flúor
gargle	la gárgara
glasses	los anteojos, gafas
graft	el injerto
heat	el calor
hormone	la hormona
humidifier	un humedificador
ice	el hielo
immunization	la inmunización
injection	la inyección
insulin	la insulina
iodine	el yodo
iron	el hierro
IUD	el dispositivo intrauterino
laxative	el laxante
liquid	líquido
lotion	la loción
lozenge	la pastilla de chupar
lumbar puncture	punción lumbar
medicine	la medicina
mineral	el mineral
needle	la aguja
nebulizer	la nebulización
oil	el aceite
ointment	el ungüento
operation	la operación
oxygen	el oxígeno
pill	la pastilla
"the pill"	la píldora (anticonceptiva)
powder	el polvo
prenatal care	cuidado prenatal
prescription	la receta
protein	proteína
sample	la muestra
soap	el jabón
stitch	el punto
suppository	el supositorio
vaginal suppository	supositorio vaginal
surgery	la cirugía
suture	la sutura

syrup	el jarabe
tablet	la tableta
test	la prueba
therapy	la terapia
transfusion	la transfusión
transplant	el transplante
treatment	el tratamiento
vaccine	la vacuna
vitamin	la vitamina
wheelchair	la silla de ruedas

9. Miscellaneous Words

animal	el animal
appetite	el apetito
ball	la pelota
basketball	la pelota de basket
beach	la playa
beer	cerveza
birthday	el cumpleaños
book	el libro
breakfast	el desayuno
cake	el pastel
candy	el dulce, caramelo
car seat	una silla para niños en el carro
cat	gata/o
cigarettes	los cigarrillos
class	la clase
condoms	los condones
contact lenses	los lentes de contacto
cookie	la galleta
cry	llorar
diapers	pañales
dinner	la cena
dog	el perro
doll	la muñeca
drugs	drogas
echocardiogram	ecocardiograma
EKG	el electrocardiograma
energy	la energía
football	el fútbol americano
friend	el/la amigo/a
glasses	los anteojos

guns	las armas
horse	el caballo
insect bite	picadura de insecto
irritable	irritable
itch	picazón, escozor
lake	el lago
lead	el plomo
library	la biblioteca
liquor	licor
lunch	el almuerzo
party	la fiesta
period	el período
pet	la mascota
play	jugar
playground	el patio de recreo
rollerskate	patinar
sad	triste
school	la escuela
seat belt	el cinturón de seguridad
shiver	tiritar
skateboard	el patinete
soccer	el futból
sports	el deporte
swim	nadar
swimming pool	piscina
teacher	el/la maestro/a
team	el equipo
thermometer	el termómetro
toy	el juguete
ultrasound	ultrasonido
vacation	las vacaciones
vision	la vista
wine	vino
X-ray	rayos X
zoo	el zoológico

Recommended Childhood Immunization Schedule
United States, 2002

Age ▶ Vaccine ▼	Birth	1 mo	2 mos	4 mos	6 mos	12 mos	15 mos	18 mos	24 mos	4-6 yrs	11-12 yrs	13-18 yrs
Hepatitis B[1]	Hep B #1 only if mother HBsAg(-)											
		Hep B #2			Hep B #3						Hep B series	
Diphtheria, Tetanus, Pertussis[2]			DTaP	DTaP	DTaP		DTaP			DTaP	Td	
Haemophilus influenzae type b[3]			Hib	Hib	Hib	Hib						
Inactivated Polio[4]			IPV	IPV		IPV				IPV		
Measles, Mumps, Rubella[5]						MMR #1				MMR #2	MMR #2	
Varicella[6]						Varicella				Varicella		
Pneumococcal[7]			PCV	PCV	PCV	PCV			PCV	PPV		
Hepatitis A[8]										Hepatitis A series		
Influenza[9]						Influenza (yearly)						

Vaccines below this line are for selected populations

range of recommended ages — catch-up vaccination — preadolescent assessment

This schedule indicates the recommended ages for routine administration of currently licensed childhood vaccines, as of December 1, 2001, for children through age 18 years. Any dose not given at the recommended age should be given at any subsequent visit when indicated and feasible. Indicates age groups that warrant special effort to administer those vaccines not previously given. Additional vaccines may be licensed and recommended during the year. Licensed combination vaccines may be used whenever any components of the combination are indicated and the vaccine's other components are not contraindicated. Providers should consult the manufacturers' package inserts for detailed recommendations.

Approved by the Advisory Committee on Immunization Practices (www.cdc.gov/nip/acip), the American Academy of Pediatrics (www.aap.org), and the American Academy of Family Physicians (www.aafp.org).

(continued on page 210)

1. **Hepatitis B vaccine (Hep B).** All infants should receive the first dose of hepatitis B vaccine soon after birth and before hospital discharge; the first dose may also be given by age 2 months if the infant's mother is HBsAg-negative. Only monovalent hepatitis B vaccine can be used for the birth dose. Monovalent or combination vaccine containing hepatitis B may be used to complete the series; 4 doses of vaccine may be administered if combination vaccine is used. The second dose should be given at least 4 weeks after the first dose, except for Hib-containing vaccine which cannot be administered before age 6 weeks. The third dose should be given at least 16 weeks after the first dose and at least 8 weeks after the second dose. The last dose in the vaccination series (third or fourth dose) should not be administered before age 6 months.

   Infants born to HBsAg-positive mothers should receive hepatitis B vaccine and 0.5 mL hepatitis B immune globulin (HBIG) within 12 hours of birth at separate sites. The second dose is recommended at age 1-2 months and the vaccination series should be completed (third or fourth dose) at age 6 months.

   Infants born to mothers whose HBsAg status is unknown should receive the first dose of the hepatitis B vaccine series within 12 hours of birth. Maternal blood should be drawn at the time of delivery to determine the mother's HBsAg status; if the HBsAg test is positive, the infant should receive HBIG as soon as possible (no later than age 1 week).

2. **Diphtheria and tetanus toxoids and acellular pertussis vaccine (DTaP).** The fourth dose of DTaP may be administered as early as age 12 months, provided 6 months have elapsed since the third dose and the child is unlikely to return at age 15-18 months. **Tetanus and diphtheria toxoids (Td)** is recommended at age 11-12 years if at least 5 years have elapsed since the last dose of tetanus and diphtheria toxoid-containing vaccine. Subsequent routine Td boosters are recommended every 10 years.

3. ***Haemophilus influenzae* type b (Hib) conjugate vaccine.** Three Hib conjugate vaccines are licensed for infant use. If PRP-OMP (PedvaxHIB® or ComVax® [Merck]) is administered at ages 2 and 4 months, a dose at age 6 months is not required. DTaP/Hib combination products should not be used for primary immunization in infants at ages 2, 4 or 6 months, but can be used as boosters following any Hib vaccine.

4. **Inactivated polio vaccine (IPV).** An all-IPV schedule is recommended for routine childhood polio vaccination in the United States. All children should receive 4 doses of IPV at ages 2 months, 4 months, 6-18 months, and 4-6 years.

5. **Measles, mumps, and rubella vaccine (MMR).** The second dose of MMR is recommended routinely at age 4-6 years but may be administered during any visit, provided at least 4 weeks have elapsed since the first dose and that both doses are administered beginning at or after age 12 months. Those who have not previously received the second dose should complete the schedule by the 11-12 year old visit.

6. **Varicella vaccine.** Varicella vaccine is recommended at any visit at or after age 12 months for susceptible children, ie, those who lack a reliable history of chickenpox. Susceptible persons aged ≥13 years should receive 2 doses, given at least 4 weeks apart.

7. **Pneumococcal vaccine.** The heptavalent **pneumococcal conjugate vaccine (PCV)** is recommended for all children age 2-23 months. It is also recommended for certain children age 24-59 months. **Pneumococcal polysaccharide vaccine (PPV)** is recommended in addition to PCV for certain high-risk groups. See *MMWR* 2000;49(RR-9):1-35.

8. **Hepatitis A vaccine.** Hepatitis A vaccine is recommended for use in selected states and regions, and for certain high-risk groups; consult your local public health authority. See *MMWR* 1999;48(RR-12);1-37.

9. **Influenza vaccine.** Influenza vaccine is recommended annually for children age ≥6 months with certain risk factors (including but not limited to asthma, cardiac disease, sickle cell disease, HIV, diabetes; see *MMWR* 2001;50:(RR-4):1-44), and can be administered to all others wishing to obtain immunity. Children aged ≤12 years should receive vaccine in a dosage appropriate for their age (0.25 mL if age 6-35 months or 0.5 mL if aged ≥3 years). Children aged ≤8 years who are receiving influenza vaccine for the first time should be separated by at least 4 weeks.

For additional information about vaccines, vaccine supply, and contraindications for immunization, please visit the National Immunization Program Web site at www.cdc.gov/nip or call the National Immunization Hotline at 800/232-2522 (English) or 800/232-0233 (Spanish).

Index

212